C000154016

RAW
PERFECTION

Sculpt Your Body
Enhance Your Mind
Revolutionise Your Life

Mike Nash
www.rawperfection.co.uk

DISCLAIMER

The information within these pages is not intended to replace medical advice or be a substitute for a physician. But remember, doctors are not robots. I'm sure you've had bad experiences with some doctors and good experiences with others. Find a helpful one. Find one that wants you to succeed and cares about your health. Find one that is knowledgeable in the area of nutrition and health. That's your responsibility.

If you are currently taking a course of prescription medication, you should never alter your eating habits without consulting your doctor or specialist because dietary changes usually affect the metabolism of prescription drugs, especially if you are taking medication for a diabetic condition. Because there is always some risk involved, the author, publisher, and/or distributors of this book are not responsible for any adverse detoxification effects or consequences resulting from the use of any suggestions or procedures described hereafter.

Some of the devices/mind-machines and procedures described in RAW PERFECTION are experimental. Conclusive studies of the long and short-term effects of some of these devices/mind-machines and procedures have not been performed. None of the information contained in this book should be construed as a claim or representation that these devices are intended for the use in the diagnosis, cure, treatment, or prevention of disease or any other medical condition. The use of some of these devices may be dangerous for those who are not in sound mental and physical health. For example, the light and sound devices that use flickering light may produce seizures in those subject to photo-induced epilepsy. Anyone taking or withdrawing from prescription or recreational drugs should be aware that drug use may affect his or her perceptions and responses to the stimuli of some of these devices. Some of the devices are restricted by law to use under medical supervision only. Before using these instruments consult your physician and check with your federal, state and local regulatory agencies for general advice.

Published by Raw Perfection Ltd. Milton Keynes, England
Copyright ©Philip Michael Nash 2002
Produced in England by Print Solutions Partnership, Surrey, England
Photography by Annette Reed
Cover design by Sharon Holdstock – www.shazzie.com

ISBN 0-9542271-0-7

British Library Cataloguing in Publication Data.
A catalogue record for this book is available from the British Library.

All rights reserved. No part of this publication may be reproduced, stored in a retrieval system, or transmitted, in any form or by any means, electronic, mechanical, photocopying, recording or otherwise, without the prior permission of the publishers.

This book is dedicated to Alan Austin-Smith, friend, mentor and founder of Take Control and the Success Scholarship. Without his commitment to helping others realise their full potential, this book would never have been written. Thank-you Alan.

ACKNOWLEDGEMENTS

The actual writing of RAW PERFECTION came from a journey that started when I was 17 and will probably never end. My first thank you goes to my dad Anthony Nash who introduced me to 'The 7 Habits of Highly Effective People' by Stephen Covey, and 'Unlimited Power' by Anthony Robbins. I attended Anthony Robbins' three day 'Fear Into Power – Firewalk' experience on my eighteenth birthday and really never looked back. Anthony Robbins inspired me to do my best to make the world a better place. I'm sure RAW PERFECTION will do just that.

Seminars with Richard Bandler, Paul Mckenna and Michael Breen of McKennaBreen Ltd allowed me to learn a great deal about NLP and Hypnosis, but more importantly allowed me to meet Alan Austin-Smith, creator of 'Take Control' and 'The Success Scholarship'. By working with Alan I learned to 'live the dream' and not just dream about it. That was four years ago. Since then I've worked full time in a variety of jobs and isolated myself off from most of the world in order to finish this book. RAW PERFECTION will change the world in a better way and I acknowledge those who showed up at just the right time to help me push it forward.

Special thanks go to Annette Reed for her photos used for the cover and for her early opinions of various chapters. To David Wolfe, Stephen Arlin and Karon Knowler for their passion in the area of 'raw foodism' and especially to Sharon Holdstock for designing the cover of RAW PERFECTION and for proof-reading the entire text. Finally to the love of my life Emma Goodridge for reading the final version and spotting even more errors, whilst our baby, Charlie Nash, cried out for food! Also thanks goes out to my mum. If I didn't mention her, there would be hell to pay!

PREPARE YOURSELF...

CONTENTS

NOTE TO READER

Throughout RAW PERFECTION, I talk of a perfect diet and various lifestyle changes that are necessary to achieve amazing results from the principles within this book. Although the changes I recommend are very definite and clearly defined, I don't expect you to master them overnight, and neither should you try to. RAW PERFECTION is a journey, not a destination. I wrote this book out of a desire to use food and other powerful principles to enhance my energy and the way I feel, and therefore revolutionise my life. When I'm feeling ecstatic and energetic my life is awesome, and obviously I want this state every minute of every day. If you only apply 10% of what you are about to read you'll make very noticeable gains in the area of health and vitality. The more you apply the better the results. The only reason I refer to 'perfection' is to give you a reference of what it takes to create 'explosive' health and 'monumental' vitality. The closer you get to this standard, the easier and more fulfilling your life will become – but it won't happen overnight. It has taken me over seven years to find what works for me.

In my naive youth I experimented with recreation drugs, (something I hope you never do) but can tell you from the bottom of my heart that the 'high' I experience from the principles of RAW PERFECTION is more powerful, more joyous and more blissful than any drug, and there is no 'come down'!

A word of warning though, RAW PERFECTION is very powerful. You need to read it from cover to cover to ensure you understand how each and every principle inter-relates.

The first approach to mastering RAW PERFECTION is to dive straight in and head for perfection, but I suggest you steer clear of this approach! If you decide to alter your eating patterns abruptly, beware! By doing so you may invite the symptoms of severe detoxification. Tread carefully.

The second approach is to gradually make a transition. The process of detoxification will be less intense and will last longer. I spent many years making the transition to a 100% raw diet and found myself reverting back to old habits time after time. That's life! Embrace it, recognise it, and above all, welcome it! It will happen, you will have your 'off days' but by reading and understanding the principles of RAW PERFECTION you'll have a proven plan to get back on the path to scintillating health... and stay there!

YOU HAVE THE POWER TO SUCCEED ARE YOU GOING TO USE IT?

When I began writing RAW PERFECTION, it was my mission to seek out the most effective principles in the areas of health, nutrition and peak performance, and fuse them together to create an approach unlike any other. I wanted to create a program that delivered so many distinctions and nutritional wisdom it would raise the standards of health to a whole new level. In my mind, RAW PERFECTION had to become the most powerful and effective system the world had ever seen! I wanted to help everyone from the individual striving to win Olympic gold to the millions of people wanting to lose a few pounds of unwanted flab.

Many authors claim that the process of writing a book is 20% inspiration and 80% perspiration. I couldn't agree more! In the four years it took to perfect what you're holding right now, I spent countless hours writing, researching, re-writing and editing.

Every writer knows how frustrating it can be to complete a chapter, or even finish a book. Many say that a book is never truly finished, but abandoned by the author when they've had enough of writing it! In my case this isn't true. I have made it my personal mission to bring to you the finest, most unique, tried and tested methods for producing revolutionary change on every level and now that it's complete, I'm more inspired about RAW PERFECTION than ever before!

LET THE JOURNEY BEGIN...

RAW PERFECTION leaves no stone unturned. In fact, I haven't yet found a book that delivers so much powerful information, on so many seemingly diverse subjects, and ties them together so beautifully. No other book that I've read combines the subjects of peak performance nutrition, hormonal control, stress, exercise, mind enhancing technology and longevity, as perfectly as the one you hold in your hands, and when you master it, you'll see why!

You've a lot to look forward to, so get excited. I'll share with you exactly what it takes to be in *total* control and you'll soon realise, like many thousands before you, a few simple distinctions can truly change your life forever.

THE FIRST STEP TO RAW PERFECTION: A POWERFUL STATE OF MIND

If you want to succeed, you'll need to condition two states of mind. The first is desire. A desire to learn the tools and strategies that are at the leading edge of nutrition and peak performance, a desire to break through any challenges that may prevent you from being all that you can be, and a desire to revolutionise your life. The second state is commitment. A commitment to work through the 'gold-mine' of ideas and concepts that can be found in each of the powerful chapters that await you. A commitment to follow through and tackle the challenges you're likely to face and a commitment to do whatever it takes to succeed. By simply reading this book from cover to cover, you'll expose yourself to the most successful life-enhancing principles in existence! Whether you want an amazingly efficient digestive system or control over the key hormones that determine the quality of your health, RAW PERFECTION delivers. In as little as two months you could be looking in the mirror at a 'new you', astonished at how much you've learnt and applied. You'll see the results for yourself, but more importantly, you'll feel them...everywhere!

RE-IGNITING THE LONG FORGOTTEN DREAM

Follow the simple principles within these pages and your dream of having perfect health and a perfect figure will soon become part of your daily reality. Remember, the quality of your health and the quality of your life isn't a question of capability, you are capable of incredible things. Sometimes however you may have failed to tap your full potential. It's my goal to challenge you. First to take control of your immediate future and secondly to help you condition the habits that will secure your success.

Just stop for a moment and think about your current eating habits. Do you jump out of bed in the morning and like a detective, seek out the foods that positively affect the functioning of your brain and nervous system? Or... Do you lazily roll out of bed, stumble down the stairs and head straight for the coffee? Whatever your life is like at the moment, there is room for improvement. It doesn't matter if you want to lose 400lbs or 4lbs, whether you want to win Olympic gold or perform more energetically at the gym, if you make the decision to excel, everything you've ever dreamt of will be in your reach. Just remember one thing...

SUCCESS OR FAILURE DOESN'T HAPPEN OVERNIGHT

Success happens one step at a time, one day at a time, and is dependent on how committed you are to making incremental improvements. The same is true with the material in this book. **If you want success you must master each of the following principles individually until you are able to see how they create the ultimate approach I call RAW PERFECTION.** Many approaches to health fail because the author concentrates on one principle alone, leading their followers into a false sense of certainty that 'their way is the only way'. I believe RAW PERFECTION will set you free from such a limited mindset. RAW PERFECTION will share with you key principles that have proven successful since the beginning of time. It's up to you to then create the daily habits that will determine your success. I've had to discover what works for me and I'll give you many clues as to what is likely to work for you. Gradually you'll expand your mind and join the elite group of people who are free from disease, living longer, and turning back the hands of time. The last key to the winning formula is simple...

RESPONSIBILITY: THE ONLY WAY FORWARD

When you take responsibility you'll search for the answers that will cause you to succeed. When you take responsibility you'll find role models of success in the areas you want to master. When you take responsibility you'll only have yourself to answer to if things don't go according to plan. Maybe you'll book an appointment with your doctor before you begin to make powerful changes to your diet and your health. (If you take any drugs – prescription or non-prescription – or have been recently, I recommend you see your physician because dietary changes can effect the metabolism of prescription drugs). Maybe you'll read other books before you begin your quest to a more fulfilling life. Whatever your choice, by taking responsibility, you'll be taking action – action that will set in motion a chain of events that will ultimately shape your destiny.

THE RAW PERFECTION MENTALITY WILL SET YOU FREE

If you've ever asked the question 'How can I lose weight and keep it off' you're reading the right book. But from now on, forget about weight loss and focus entirely on 'optimal body function'. What good is weight loss if your body isn't operating at it's best? What good is weight loss if your brain isn't functioning more coherently? What good is weight loss if you don't have control over the production of various hormones within your body? What good is weight loss if you run your enzyme supply down to a level that can damage your health? You'll understand more about these concepts later, for now, ask a different quality of question:

♦ How can I influence my body and its systems to operate with laser-like precision and uncanny efficiency, whilst my body remains lean and operating at its best?

Your aim is to learn the most cutting edge strategies to get your body working as perfectly as possible. That is where we are headed. A word of warning though. To opt out of the eating habits of the herd does require a certain degree of self-discipline. People will challenge you and your new habits for many reasons, but as long as you refer to the end of each chapter and refresh your knowledge continuously, you'll have every reason to continue and succeed. Changing the habits of a lifetime can be easy if you have enough reasons to begin. That is the power of RAW PERFECTION. Each principle builds upon the last creating an almost magical approach to health. This is my ultimate goal for you, to see food as a source of pleasure, which it is, and always will be, but also as the ultimate controller of your mind/body and emotions. With the right foods you unlock the door to more than just optimal health. Some people have talked about being so highly 'charged' with energy that they've felt more connected to their religion or spiritual path. Whether this happens to you or not remains to be seen, but the kind of energy I'm talking about can only be built on a foundation of superior eating habits and superior lifestyle habits…

IN SEARCH OF PERFECTION: UNLEASHING THE AWESOME POWER OF YOUR RETICULAR ACTIVATING SYSTEM (RAS)

If you keep your focus on perfection and being the very best you can possibly be, something magical will happen. You'll mysteriously find yourself gravitating towards anything and everything that can help you achieve your goals. Why? Because of a unique part of your brain called your Reticular Activating System (RAS). Your RAS simply determines what you notice and what you pay attention to. It is responsible for the screening of data into your mind. You see…as you are sitting there now…reading this book…there are countless pieces of information you could focus on…you could focus on the temperature of your left toe…or the tightness of the clothes you are wearing …or you could focus on the sounds around you and how they are affecting you…you may even focus entirely on the words you are reading…or the whiteness of the page…as you read.

You are constantly being bombarded by infinite amounts of data, and because your conscious mind can only focus on a limited number of elements at any one time, your brain has to decide what to delete. It has to decide what *not* to pay attention to. It does this by focusing on what you believe to be of importance, whilst ignoring the irrelevant. This is where your RAS comes in. If you buy a new item of clothing or a car for example, don't you find that you begin to see it everywhere! Do you think it didn't exist before? Of course not! The reality is that it probably did, you just weren't paying attention. Your RAS wasn't sensitised to its existence.

Now, when you focus entirely on perfection and being the best you can be, your brain will delete all the information that isn't necessary for the attainment of your goal, and highlight what you need to know in order to fully succeed. Be specific. Start now by making a mental image of what you'll look like and be like once you've achieved your goals. See yourself having finished reading RAW PERFECTION. See yourself applying all the principles successfully and easily. See yourself the way you want. Make the picture big and bright and appealing so that you feel a burning desire to do everything you can to become what you see. Let yourself know how much energy you want, what time you want to wake up in the morning and how you want to feel. Let yourself know that you want to squeeze the maximum amount of juice out of your life whilst enjoying every minute. The more appealing you make this image, the easier it will be for your brain to highlight what you need to do in order to achieve this kind of success. By doing this you'll begin to notice everything around you that can assist you. People will start showing up that can assist you in your quest, articles in magazines may reinforce something you are about to learn and before long you may start meeting people that have also read this book and can share with you their own experiences. I know this may seem like a strange way of thinking, but by the time you finish RAW PERFECTION it'll make perfect sense.

WHAT YOU ARE ABOUT TO LEARN WILL CHANGE THE WAY YOU PERCIEVE FOOD FOREVER

Before long, an apple won't just be an apple, but a source of phytochemicals, vitamins, minerals, pectin, enzymes and fibre. You'll think of it as something that cannot only help control your blood sugar levels because of it's low rating on the glycemic index (see appendix 3), but you'll also appreciate that with its high water/mineral content it will help maintain the acid/alkaline balance in your body, whilst assisting in maximising your elimination cycle. An avocado won't just be something you can make guacamole from, but an insulin decreasing hormonal delight that supplies an abundance of essential oils helping to build powerful hormone-like substances within your body known as eicosanoids. Your RAS is responsible for pointing you in the direction you want to go. Just take a look at the people that seem to spend their whole life focusing on foods that are low in fat. When they go into the supermarket, that is all they see! Their RAS is sensitised to them, but who says that low-fat food is healthy? Did you know that certain types of fat are as critical to your health as vitamins and minerals? In fact, by not including certain fats in your diet, you are guaranteeing sub-optimum nutrition, whilst opening the door to illness and disease. Many diets limit what you can eat, restricting your choice, but rather than taking anything away, RAW PERFECTION gives you...

FREEDOM: EXPANDING YOUR CHOICE AND FLEXIBILITY

What you are about to learn is how food effects your body with laser-like precision. With your new level of understanding and knowledge you'll be so motivated to eat foods that assist your health, energy and life, there will be no room for any other option. You'll begin to learn about how *you* function at *your* best and how to optimise *your* body function.

FOOD: THE MOST POWERFUL DRUG KNOWN TO MANKIND

Every time you eat or drink something you give your body a very powerful set of highly specific instructions. Your biochemistry changes to accommodate what you've put in your system and your hormonal responses adjust accordingly. The same happens when you take a prescription from a doctor. When you swallow a pill or a medicine, your body has a response to the medication, just as it does to food.

Remember there is one prescription you must follow for the rest of your life if you want to thrive. Get plenty of sunlight, breath as much fresh air as you can, drink plenty of fresh filtered water and understand and use food as if it was a prescription drug. It has incredible power over your physiology. It's up to you to discover what makes food so powerful, otherwise ignorance will catch up with you! Food is your prescription for life. Use the prescription wisely and you'll succeed beyond your wildest dreams. Use it sloppily and you may wake up one day in hospital, in a state of very poor health, knocking at death's door, regretting your decision. It's that simple!

NO DIET SYSTEM IS PERFECT, BUT YOU ARE!

RAW PERFECTION is a personal science. It's up to you to use each and every life-enhancing principle to create an incredible life, and the only way to do this is to learn how the principles work synergistically, and commit to constant and never ending improvement. This is what mastery is all about – Putting you in the driving seat and letting you take control.

I've spent over a decade working in the fitness industry, becoming an expert in hypnosis and N.L.P. and working successfully as a training consultant with hundreds of people from all walks of life. I want you to know that I've made it my commitment to learn what it takes to massively impact my life and now I'm going to share these 'secrets' with *you*, to ensure *your* success.

Once you've read RAW PERFECTION in its entirety, you'll find the best way to organise these principles so that YOU benefit. And to me, YOU are the only one who matters; YOU are the only one who knows when YOU feel excellent.

ARE YOU READY FOR THE CHALLENGE?

Two weeks of following the principles of RAW PERFECTION should excite you. Take a look why:

1. **Razor sharp thinking and pure mental clarity**. As you begin to maintain tight control of your blood sugar levels, you'll find yourself developing laser-like concentration as you wave good-bye to the mental haziness associated with the high carbohydrate diet. Afternoon mental slumps will be a thing of the past.
2. **Unlimited energy and vibrancy**. As you begin to appreciate the role of chlorophyll-rich foods and their powerful balancing effects, you'll begin to rebuild your blood and rebalance your body. How would you like to feel more refreshed and alert in the morning and more energised throughout the day?
3. **Look in the mirror with admiration as your shape changes before your very eyes.** Don't expect to shed all of your excess weight in the first week! But do expect to lose about 1 to 2 pounds of fat and about 2 to 3 pounds of retained water. A week from now you could be 5 or more pounds lighter. You'll have control over your insulin levels (an excess of which can cause water retention) and be more balanced hormonally. Then it will only be a matter of time before you develop the body of your dreams!

4. **Connect with your deepest feelings of wellbeing, joy and vibrancy**. Violent blood-sugar fluctuations cause people to feel tired, moody, hungry and irritable. A week from now however, you can feel more balanced, more in control and more motivated. Why? Because your energy will be constant. You'll feel like you are cruising through choppy seas in an ocean liner, rather than a rickety old raft!

5. **Eliminate carbohydrate cravings**. RAW PERFECTION will motivate you to eat foods that are so nutrient dense, you won't even need supplements. In the process you'll automatically consume fewer calories yet experience less cravings as you meet all your nutritional needs. Once you've taken care of that, you can concentrate on the exciting new ways you are going to use your newfound energy!

6. **Fine-tune your insulin levels**. You'll learn shortly how the over-stimulation of insulin can destroy your body, leading to obesity, diabetes and heart disease. Fortunately, recent studies from Harvard medical school have shown that by eating in accordance with the principles of hormonal control, insulin-controlling benefits kick in almost immediately.

7. **Eliminate stress and embrace a powerful mind.** In the final section, once you've mastered the basics and find yourself crackling with energy and incredibly motivated, you'll learn how to use your motivation and energy in ways that enhance your brain and revolutionise your life.

That's all I have to say for now. Let's get down to business and journey together through the magical land of RAW PERFECTION. Have fun, experiment like never before and maybe one day we'll get the chance to meet each other.

PART ONE

BUILDING AN UNSHAKEABLE FOUNDATION

CHAPTER 1

NATURE'S FIRST LAW: RAW POWER

Sit back. Take a deep breath and relax. Imagine yourself in the future. You feel different. You feel more alive. You feel like you did when you were a child, full of zest and vitality, but the feeling is more powerful. You feel as if you've somehow been granted perfect health. You look in the mirror and notice a body that is slim and firm. You look closely at your skin and find it hard to find a single blemish. Your hair is rich and full. Your eyes twinkle and sparkle and you feel incredible!

As your bloodstream crackles with electricity, your immune system effortlessly destroys foreign invaders. Every part of your being is working beautifully and in harmony like the philharmonic orchestra. Your life seems effortless and blissfully joyful, and your mind is full of good humour and joy!

The future can be inspiring, can't it? But the future isn't somewhere you go, it is a place you create from the decisions you make every moment of every day.

ACCEPT NATURE'S LAW AND
ADOPT THE MINDSET OF A CHAMPION

If you want exceptional health, you must eat exceptional foods. Take a look at nature and you'll see exceptional foods everywhere. Exceptional foods rebuild your body and mind, leading you down a road to an amazing future. Everything your body is made of was once the air you breathed, the water you drank, and most importantly the food you ate. The colloidal mineral structure of your body is built out of the foods that have passed your lips. Any simple change to your nutrition habits will alter the look and function of your body and brain. Hunt out and eat the finest foods available and you'll dramatically improve the foundation upon which your body is built.

COMMON SENSE SEPARATES TRUTH FROM FICTION

If you want to destroy something, set fire to it! If you want to destroy the vital elements within any food, cook it! When you heat any fruit, vegetable or plant food, you began to breakdown its natural structure. The more heat - the more destruction! Fire completely destroys. No food can be improved when heat is added. Cooking kills!

♦ Temperatures of 118 degrees Fahrenheit or more destroy critical enzymes within food. The result: Cooked food isn't completely broken down by your body and travels, undigested, into your small intestine, where it putrefies, poisoning your blood. Enzymes are critical to life and need to be present within food for optimal digestion.
♦ Cooking leaches minerals out of food. Nobody has studied the effect of minerals as extensively as Dr. Joel Wallach. He has performed 17500 autopsies on 454 species and on 3000 humans and has proved they all died of some sort of mineral deficiency. He was nominated in 1991 for the Nobel Prize in Medicine.
♦ Cooking also destroys vitamins, which are needed to control the absorption and use of minerals.
♦ Whenever fat is cooked, transfatty acids are produced. Transfatty acids are one of the most destructive elements of any cooked food diet. They decrease testosterone, increase abnormal sperm, and interfere with pregnant animals. They are a major source of damaging

free radicals and research shows that cooks who spend time wok or pan-frying have a higher incidence of lung cancer.

♦ When you eat cooked food, your body has to release copious amounts of enzymes in order to break down the food. Without enzymes, your food would never digest. Your enzyme supply is limited and cooked food runs it down to dangerously low levels.

Although I'm sure you're shocked at what you've just read, I'm not expecting you to immediately eliminate all cooked food from your diet. What I do want you do to is begin considering the importance of raw plant foods. Raw plant foods are easily digested, and within only 24-36 hours pass easily through your digestive tract. Cooked/dead foods in comparison take 40-100+ hours and clog your system.

One research group found that people who ate a lot of fibre – via raw fruits and vegetables – excreted more calories each day compared to those eating a diet of cooked foods with the same caloric content but without the fibre.

HUMANITIES MOST IMPORTANT BATTLE:
RAW FOOD VERSUS COOKED FOOD

In their book Goldot, Lewis E. Cook Jr. and Junko Yasui recount a very powerful study. The study was performed on three groups of rats and the results were fascinating. Take a look for yourself before you come to the same conclusions as the researchers.

GROUP ONE

From birth, the first group of rats were fed a raw diet of fruits, vegetables, nuts, and whole grains. As they grew they experienced every sign of good health. They grew fast. They had strong bodies. They were free from disease. They were also free from excess fat. They reproduced with vigour and enthusiasm and paved the way for their healthy offspring. They were vivacious, spirited, and very affectionate to one another. As soon as they reached the equivalent of 80 human years they were put to sleep and autopsied. Researchers found that every organ, every gland, and every tissue was in perfect condition. A diet of raw food prevented them from experiencing the 'normal' signs of ageing and degeneration.

GROUP TWO

From birth, this group of rats was fed a diet of cooked foods: Milk, meat, white bread, soda, sweets, cakes, vitamins and medicines. As they grew they experienced many of the same diseases that afflict people in present day society such as colds, fevers, pneumonia, poor eyesight, cataracts, heart disease, arthritis, cancer, etc. But it wasn't just their biological health that was on the line. Their emotional health was also very unstable. They attacked each other consistently. They gave birth to offspring that were constantly ill, and aggressive. Death came prematurely to this group from diseases or various epidemics that swept through the entire colony. Autopsies revealed extensive degeneration to every organ, every gland, and every tissue of their bodies. The researchers had found a very impressive way to accelerate the speed in which the rats aged – by feeding them a diet similar to what most humans eat. The rats paid the ultimate price – early death from disease.

GROUP THREE

From birth, this group was fed a diet identical to Group Two until they reached an equivalent human age of 40. They displayed behavioural characteristics identical to those in the previous group and had the same poor quality of health. At the end of this 'equivalent 40 year period' the rats were placed on a strict water fast for a number of days before being introduced to a 100% raw food diet, coupled with periods of fasting. The changes were dramatic. Within one month they began showing signs of exceptional health. They became affectionate, playful and more resilient to infection, showing no signs of illness or disease. At the end of an 'equivalent 80 year period', autopsies revealed that this group had completely reversed all signs of ageing on a biological basis. Every organ, every gland, and every tissue was in perfect condition.

WARNING: YOU CANNOT IMPROVE FOOD BY COOKING IT

You hold in your hands a very powerful book, one that will shatter many illusions about health and the origins of disease. Be patient. The first step along your path is to realise that eating cooked foods has nothing to do with the normal biological requirements of your body. Fire destroys! In fact, any food that is unnecessarily heated or put to flame becomes addictive. Don't expect to break away from such habits immediately. Tread carefully. Learn. Discover. Digest. But above all, be patient and you'll find yourself on the path to the most incredible personal discovery of your life. The first part of this incredible journey is to slowly begin increasing the amount and variety of raw plant foods in your diet. For every disciplined effort in life there is a multiple reward.

THE POWER OF ENZYME RICH RAW FOOD
AND THE PERILS OF ENZYME-LESS COOKED FOOD

In the 1930s, Dr Paul Kouchakoff demonstrated that after eating cooked food, there is an increase in white blood cells in the body, a phenomenon called 'digestive leukocytosis'.

When faced with too much enzyme-less cooked food, your body will recruit white blood cells (leukocytes) to transport a large quantity of enzymes, for the task of breaking down food particles. In other words, when your body is unable to properly digest food, white blood cells will attack the food, in an effort to reduce it to usable components or eliminate it from the body. Until Kouchakoff's work, this was considered normal but Kouchakoff found that when foods are consumed in their raw state, digestive leukocytosis does not occur. Raw foods have just the right amount of natural enzymes/nutrients within them to allow them to perfectly self-digest within your digestive system. This leads to better digestion and assimilation. The message is simple:

♦ Processed food and cooked food reliably triggers off leukocyte mobilisation.
♦ Raw plant food has no such effect.

WARNING: YOUR BODY FIGHTS
COOKED FOOD LIKE A DISEASE

F.M. Pottenger conducted a 10-year study on the effect of a cooked food diet on an animal's life cycle. Pottenger raised a colony of 900 cats placed on controlled diets. He fed them only meat and milk, either raw or cooked. Those fed on raw food produced healthy kittens every year without fail. Those fed on the cooked version of the exact same food developed the same diseases which afflict humanity, including heart disease, cancer, osteoporosis, sexual impotency, paralysis, pneumonia, glandular malfunctioning, kidney disease, arthritis, difficulty in labour and severe irritability. Take a look at what happened to each generation of cats fed on the cooked food diet:

1. The first generation of kittens were ill and abnormal.
2. The second generation was born either already diseased or dead.
3. The mothers of the third generation were sterile.

Pottenger discovered that the damage created by cooked food requires four generations of raw foodism to correct. The faeces produced by the cats eating a cooked food diet caused plants to become stunted and weak. The faeces produced by the cats eating a raw food diet caused plants to grow normally. Cooked food addiction has a long-lasting effect on the future generation of our planet.

WARNING: COOKED FOOD CAUSES YOUR ORGANS TO WORK FIVE TIMES THEIR NORMAL CAPACITY AND EXHAUST PREMATURELY

It's about time more and more people questioned the use of cooked food in their diet, including you. You don't have to eliminate it immediately, but at least suspend your beliefs long enough to learn about the power of raw foods and experiment with them. Once you realise why raw foods are so powerful, through knowledge and experience, you'll understand why cooked foods have no use in your body, other than to satisfy addiction!

BEGINNING THE ULTIMATE BALANCING ACT

If raw plant foods are going to take pride of place in your diet, you're probably wondering where to start, how to keep variety in your diet and how to make it easy. The answer to all these questions will be presented to you in the next few chapters where you'll begin to discover that the only way to succeed consistently on a all raw diet learn how to balance raw plant foods correctly. This is the magic formula! Be patient. It'll be presented to you when the time is right in a future chapter...

LOOKING TO THE FUTURE WITH A GLINT IN YOUR EYE

It's up to you whether you choose to eat a 100% raw food diet or not, but as long as you continue to increase the amount of raw food in your diet you'll be making progress. The closer you are to 100% the closer you are to nature's intention! But the all-important factor is how you build the raw portion of your diet. This is where the magic formula comes in. With the magic formula, you'll discover:

♦ How to use raw plant food to supply maximum nutrition with the minimum amount of food.
♦ How to balance the key hormones of your body and maximise fat loss.
♦ How to decrease stress hormones and enhance youth accelerating hormones.
♦ How to optimise neurotransmitter equilibrium within your brain, fostering a more alert, vibrant state of mind.
♦ How to burn parasites out of your body.
♦ How to restore a balanced internal flora encouraging optimal digestion.
♦ How to prevent cravings, maximising the life and vitality of every cell in your body.

Without this magic formula you may be vegetarian/vegan and still suffer from blood-sugar abnormalities, cravings for cooked foods and cravings for high sugary foods. More about this later. For now consider this...

MAXIMISE NUTRIENT UPTAKE WITH RAW-GANIC FOOD

Never question the power of raw organic plant food! Back in 1993, Bob Smith, a trace minerals laboratory analyst began purchasing samples of both organic and commercial plant foods. He wanted to know why organic foods were getting so much attention, and if that attention was warranted. For over two years he studied each of his samples for trace elements. Take a look at his conclusions and decide for yourself whether raw organic plant food should take pride of place in your diet:

1. Organically grown pears had two to nearly three times more chromium, iodine, manganese, molybdenum, silicon, and zinc.
2. Organically grown corn had twenty times more calcium and manganese, and two to five times more copper, magnesium, molybdenum, selenium and zinc.

3. Organically grown wheat had twice the calcium, four times more magnesium, five times more manganese, and 13 times more selenium than the commercial wheat.
4. Organically grown potatoes had two or more times the boron, selenium, silicon, strontium, and sulphur, and 60% more zinc.

His other findings were that organic foods also had lower quantities of toxic trace elements, such as aluminium, lead, and mercury. There's usually a section in every supermarket now where you can buy organic cooked food such as organic biscuits, crisps etc. Organic food is not enough, foods must be 'raw-ganic' if you're going to succeed.

SPICE UP YOUR FOOD AND SPICE UP YOUR LIFE

If you want to include more raw plant food in your diet today, remember one thing: People often have problems transitioning to a raw food diet because they haven't learnt how to spice up their dishes. The key to success is using herbs and spices to create mouth-watering dishes that tickle your taste buds and arouse your senses. From Italy to the Far East or from France to Mexico, you'll find every culture has its own preferred style and own preferred blend of herbs and spices that create distinctive textures and flavours. Begin experimenting today!

♦ Chinese: Anise, garlic, and ginger
♦ French: Bay leaves, garlic, rosemary, tarragon, and thyme
♦ Greek: Cinnamon, garlic, mint and oregano
♦ Indian: Cardamom, coriander seeds, cumin, curry, fenugreek, ginger, mustard seeds, and turmeric
♦ Italian: Basil, bay leaves, fennel seeds, garlic, marjoram, oregano, red pepper flakes, rosemary and sage
♦ Mexican: Chilli, cilantro, cinnamon, cumin, coriander, and oregano
♦ Middle eastern: Cinnamon, cumin, garlic, mint, parsley, and oregano

Herbalists know that spices can help with ailments as diverse as stomach problems, toothache and chilblains. In response to hot and spicy food, your brain produces pain-killing endorphins that promote a mini-euphoric high! More about this phenomenon later.

ARE YOU READY FOR THE CHALLENGE?

No stone is left unturned when it comes to understanding how various foods affect your magical being. Knowledge is power and this chapter is only the beginning. Start today and remember one thing. If you've spent your whole life trying to get control of your weight, or trying to get control of your health, or trying to break the barriers of a personal best in your field of endeavour, let the struggle come to a grinding halt! What you've done in the past may have had some degree of success, but what you are learning now will exhaust every avenue necessary, allowing you to become an unrivalled success. Be the best you've ever been. Now is the time and this is the book. Let your life blossom right in front of your very eyes.

Over quite a short time an all-raw, or nearly all-raw diet will generate Raw Power. Here's why:

◆ You'll begin to radiate more energy. Andre Simoneton found that we radiate more energy if we eat foods that also give off a high level of radiance. Examples are wheatgrass juice, Blue Green algae, organic fruits, organic vegetables and sprouted nuts, seeds, pulses and grains.

◆ Raw foods cleanse your body of stored wastes and toxins. These wastes interfere with the proper functioning of cells and organs and are responsible for lowering your energy.

◆ Raw foods restore optimal sodium/potassium and acid/alkaline balance. More about this later.

◆ Raw foods offer, in perfect and complementary combination, all the nutrients essential for maximum vitality at the cellular level.

◆ Raw foods increase the efficiency with which cells take up oxygen. Oxygen is necessary for cells to release energy and carry out an infinite number of critical life processes.

◆ Raw foods increase the micro-electrical potential of cells, improving your body's use of oxygen, energising your muscles and brain.

◆ You'll begin to unlock nature's pharmacy, as you tap into the unlimited storehouse of phytochemicals (plant chemicals) present within plant foods. Phytochemicals not only prevent many diseases, but virtually guarantee unrivalled health. To maximise your phytochemical intake, focus on a variety of colourful raw foods.

◆ One research group found that people who ate a lot of fibre – via raw fruits and vegetables – excreted more calories on a daily basis than those on a cooked diet of the same caloric content but without the fibre.

◆ Forget calorie counting once and for all. It is impossible to put on extra fat content by eating raw foods alone. More about this later!

◆ Raw foods prevent a build up of waste matter between the target tissue within a cell and the protective endothelial cells that are in direct contact with the bloodstream. This space, known as the interstitial space needs to be kept clear to allow optimal exchange of nutrients and hormones. More about hormones later!

◆ Did you know that the number of old cells being replaced on a day to day basis is between 300 hundred billion and 800 billion? The difference – approximately 500 billion! That's a big difference, especially if you can influence it! And the only way to prevent such dramatic losses is to eliminate cooked/processed food and replace them with raw-ganic foods.

◆ The message from this chapter is simple: There are distinct physiological differences between animals that feed exclusively on raw foods and animals that feed on cooked foods. Shouldn't they be biologically identical if both food types have the same physiological effect?

◆ If you want to begin immediately, turn to appendix 1 and find the RAW PERFECTION shopping list. Buy as many raw foods that appeal to you and begin experimenting.

Roll up your sleeves, sharpen your knives, clear space in your refrigerator for magical RAW PERFECTION foods, and let's begin. It's up to you to take action to create momentum. Begin slowly and remember, wherever you go and whatever you do, always search for foods that flood your body with zest, sparkle and spirit. The choice is yours, dead food and a lifeless body, or live raw food and a vibrant body.

THE RAW PERFECTION EVALUATION:
Do you eat a variety of colourful raw foods every day?
Do you ensure the foods you eat are delicious and mouth watering?

When you begin any life-changing program, you need momentum! You need to ensure that every action you take propels you towards unlimited success. With this kind of momentum you go far and you go fast. Let the journey begin...

CHAPTER 2

THE ACCELERATED PATH TO PARADISE HEALTH – SUPREME GREENS

Until man duplicates a blade of grass,
Nature can laugh at his so-called scientific knowledge.
– Thomas A. Edison

Whether you want to increase your strength and body mass, lose unwanted fat or increase your general health, begin loading your diet with green leafy vegetables. Constipated? – Eat more greens. Want more iron? – Eat more greens. Want more calcium – Eat more greens. Think about it, where does a cow get her calcium from for her milk? Mineral-rich green grass! I don't expect you to begin grazing in the nearest field, but I do expect you to begin seeing the magic inherent within green leafy vegetables. This chapter will open your eyes to their true power. Chlorophyll-rich foods are the blood of life and critical building blocks in the foundation of RAW PERFECTION.

NATURES MOST REMARKABLE GIFT: WHEATGRASS JUICE

Imagine a super-food so potent and so densely packed with nutrition, that it could, if it had to, supply all your nutritional requirements. Imagine a super-food teeming with essential amino acids, essential fatty acids, glucose, vitamins, minerals, phytochemicals, along with powerful blood building/cancer fighting qualities. Imagine no more. Wheatgrass juice has the power to reconstruct your body into a temple of exuberance and youth. Drink it often, and it won't be long before the air around you is crackling with electricity!

Dr. Arthur Robinson, director of the Oregon Institute of Science and Medicine credits wheatgrass as having the most preventative and restorative properties known to mankind.

In 1978 at the Linus Pauling Institute, Dr. Robinson completed a research project in which wheatgrass and live foods were fed to mice with squamos cell carcinoma (a cancer that develops in levels of the epidermis that are closer to the body's surface. They commonly appear on sun-exposed areas of the body such as the face, ear, neck, lip and back of the hands.)

Dr. Robinson's excitement was clear, "The results were spectacular. Living foods alone (including wheatgrass) decreased the incidence and severity of cancer lesions by about 75%. This result was better than that of any other nutritional program."

A PINT OF SUNSHINE PLEASE!
CHLOROPHYLL: LIQUID SUNSHINE TRANSFORMED INTO NUTRITIVE ENERGY

Chlorophyll is the green pigment in plants that allows sunlight to combine with water and carbon dioxide to form the carbohydrates that fuel your body. For our purposes, think of chlorophyll as liquid sunshine. Chlorophyll is the lifeblood of plants and the closest you'll ever get to consuming sunlight as food. In fact, when you drink chlorophyll-rich juice found in green juices such as wheatgrass juice, you get all the benefits associated with sunbathing without exposing yourself to the potentially harmful effects of direct sunlight. Wheatgrass is very cheap to grow, easy to harvest and takes no time at all to juice, each sip firing you up with solar energy.

There are many different ways you can increase the quantity of green chlorophyll-rich foods in your diet. You can blend or juice your greens making an infinite number of concoctions, or you can eat them in salads. I'll share with you some powerful practices that I use later. For now, concentrate on wheatgrass juice. It will give you the grounding you need for appreciating the healing and restorative power of green leafy vegetables. Come with me now and discover why wheatgrass can be seen as...

THE POOR MAN'S PATH TO RICHES

When compared to many of today's expensive supplements, wheatgrass is not only far superior, but easy to grow and easy to use. Simply take a handful of wheat berries, some water, a tray filled with an inch of topsoil and a cover. Within seven days at a cost of 7p a tray, you'll have enough wheatgrass to juice. Drink it daily and you'll maximise the charge of electricity around each and every one of your ten trillion cells. Wheatgrass juice is not only a superior source of chlorophyll, but also a concentrated punch of high-quality water, oxygen, enzymes, phytochemicals, carotenoids, fatty acids, trace minerals, antioxidants and amino acids. It's no wonder people who drink wheatgrass seem to stand out from the crowd, with a glint in their eye, a magic about their aura, and a spring in their stride. Wheatgrass is alive, and brings you to life in every way. It helps to release an unnatural build up of excess fats and mineral deposits. It also helps release proteins trapped in the blood, organs of digestion and organs of elimination. Every element within wheatgrass juice rushes to revitalise your entire being!

REJUVENATE YOUR BLOOD WITH CHLOROPHYLL:
GIVE YOURSELF A VIRTUAL PLANT BLOOD TRANSFUSION

Haemoglobin is the pigment that gives your blood its colour and oxygen carrying capacity. Just as haemoglobin brings life to every part of your body, chlorophyll is the pigment that brings life to plants. In 1930, Dr Hans Fisher and a group of associates won the Nobel prize, after making a groundbreaking discovery. Their work was based around the mysteries of the red blood cell. To their amazement they found that on a molecular level, the haemoglobin in human blood is practically identical to chlorophyll. The difference between the two pigments is that chlorophyll has a core of magnesium, whilst haemoglobin has a core of iron.

The resemblance between the two is so striking that:

♦ When crude chlorophyll is fed to rabbits with anaemia (low serum iron count) it restores normal red blood cell counts within approximately 15 days and is completely non toxic.
♦ A simple injection of crude chlorophyll increases red blood cell counts in healthy animals that already have normal haemoglobin levels.

USING THE POWER OF NATURE TO CURE ANAEMIA

As many as 30% of all women beyond the age of puberty in the United States may be anaemic. For men the rate of anaemia begins to increase by age fifty. The major symptoms of anaemia are fatigue and loss of appetite and these symptoms usually coincide with deficiencies of various nutrients, such as B12, folic acid, iron, copper, potassium and protein.

In 1936, research into the power of chlorophyll went one step further. Scientists J.H. Hughs and A.L. Latner of the University of Liverpool conducted some groundbreaking experiments. In their study, reported in the Journal of Physiology in 1936, they created a number of anaemic animals by bleeding them at regular intervals. Once the animals' haemoglobin levels were slashed in half, they were divided into ten different groups.

♦ Five of the groups were fed various types of chlorophyll in their diet.
♦ The other five groups of control animals were fed no chlorophyll.

The animals that received crude (raw, unrefined) chlorophyll experienced a regeneration of their blood haemoglobin levels 50% above average. In less than two weeks their blood haemoglobin levels were normal! The group receiving synthetic chlorophyll made no marked improvements, highlighting that the animal body is capable of converting *raw, unrefined* chlorophyll into haemoglobin. Synthetic versions created by decomposing natural chlorophyll and combining it with a copper ion proved to be incredibly stable, but *caused* nausea and anaemia rather than curing it!

YOU ARE ONLY AS YOUNG AS YOUR BLOOD

Dr Bernard Jensen, author of 'Chlorophyll Magic From Living Plant Food' has used green juices and wheatgrass juice to treat low serum iron counts and toxic conditions of the blood, with unrivalled success. He was able to double patients' red blood cell count in a matter of days, by prescribing 'chlorophyll water baths' and including green juices such as wheatgrass juice into their diet. If your blood is rich in iron, it will deliver more oxygen to your cells.

According to Dr Yoshihide Hagiwara research, it is the fat solubility of chlorophyll that allows it to be converted directly into haemoglobin in the lymphatic system. Chlorophyll-rich foods wake up every fibre of your being, injecting you with life and energy.

PERFORM AT YOUR BEST
IN SPITE OF DEADLY POLLUTION

It's a fact – our air, water and food is contaminated. Recent tests confirm this and the results are shocking! Many pollutants are carcinogenic, responsible for the rise in cancer, whilst others are capable of altering genes or DNA, affecting future generations. If you want to increase the strength and resistance of your body so you can co-exist with them, rather than be devastated by them, begin including an abundance of green leafy vegetables in your diet, and begin with wheatgrass juice.

A daily dose of chlorophyll, in its raw form will help protect you against the effects of radiation and the unnecessary cellular damage caused by carcinogens and other toxins. For example raw chlorophyll protects against sodium fluoride. Sodium fluoride is used as rat poison and to fluoridate drinking water. According to Dr Earp-Thomas, raw chlorophyll combines with the toxic sodium fluoride, changing its chemical composition into a safer more stable compound.

After placing a small amount of wheatgrass in a jar of regular water, to find out whether it could neutralise any of the toxins, he concluded:

"Fluorine rapidly combines with calcium phosphate and other kinetic elements to lose its toxic properties, and harden teeth and bones. That is why fresh grass would act as a catalyst to speedily change the acid fluorine into a beneficial component with a positive reaction. By using wheatgrass, which is comparatively rich in calcium phosphate, it would remove any free fluoric acid and change its negative charge to an alkaline calcium phosphate fluoride combination with a positive reaction."

For you and I, this simply means that wheatgrass has the power to simultaneously neutralise the toxic effect of fluorine, and convert it into an ally that *helps* in the maintenance of healthy bones and teeth! Whatever you decide to drink, ensure you drink up to 4oz of wheatgrass juice at least once a day!

Although there are many forms of disease, you'll learn in chapter 5 that effective health restoration always begins with detoxification. When you rid your body of unwanted waste, health begins to flourish. Wheatgrass juice acts like a detergent, purging the liver, scrubbing the intestinal tract and oxygenating blood. The elements within wheatgrass chelate and remove heavy metals from your body, highlighting it's incredible detoxifying nature. Even your faecal matter is likely to have a higher heavy metal count after you've ingested wheatgrass juice.

WHEATGRASS ENZYMES:
IT'S *NOT* THE FOOD IN YOUR LIFE
IT'S THE LIFE IN YOUR FOOD

Enzymes fire you up with incredible energy and vitality. Enzymes also detoxify harmful substances and participate in thousands of never-ending chemical changes in the body. There are two types:

1. Indogenous enzymes: These are produced naturally by your body and are incredibly powerful. Even though they are capable of great detoxification, they wear out quickly with age.
2. Exogenous enzymes: These are found in enzyme-rich fruits, vegetables and sprouts, but for a truly powerful enzyme cocktail, look no further than wheatgrass juice. If you want to spare your own enzyme supply, wheatgrass juice is the place to begin.

BANISH ACCELERATED AGEING
WITH WHEATGRASS ENZYMES

Here is a list of the most important enzymes found in wheatgrass:

- Cytochrome oxidase - Your cells will become energised with this antioxidant required for proper cell respiration.
- Lipase - Your ability to digest fat will improve with the inclusion of this fat-splitting enzyme.
- Protease - Your ability to digest and breakdown undigested protein remnants left in your digestive tract will improve as you increase the consumption of this protein digestant.
- Amylase - Your ability to digest starch will improve with the inclusion of this starch-digesting enzyme.
- Catalase and gluathione peroxide - You'll help prevent any unnecessary ageing with the inclusion of these two enzymes. They both reduce hydrogen peroxide to water before it can combine with another superoxide free radical to form the hydroxyl free radical, the most destructive of all free radicals.
- Transhydrogenase - You'll ensure a healthy heart by increasing the consumption of this enzyme since it helps in keeping the muscle tissue of the heart toned.
- Superoxide dimutase (SOD) - You'll discover the power of SOD shortly.

As you age, your body's natural production of these enzymes dwindles, reducing your ability to handle heavy fats, proteins, and excess calories. Imagine how bright your future will be as you include an early morning shot of wheatgrass juice into your routine. It'll cause your blood stream to dance and your heart to sing! The enzymes that are found in relatively high concentrations in normal red and white blood cells are cytochrome oxidase, peroxidase, and catalase, but in the body of a cancer patient these enzymes are of a dangerously low concentration. All cancer patients should include wheatgrass juice in their diets, the enzymes have been found to break down tumours and cysts.

One of the most powerful enzymes is the last enzyme on the list. Turn the page and take a look for yourself.

DRUM ROLE PLEASE!
PRESENTING THE KEY ANTI-AGEING ENZYME: SOD

Dr. Barry Halliwell, a biochemist at the University of London, Dr. M. Rister, at the University of Cologne in Germany, and Dr. Irwin Fridovich, a biochemist at Duke University have all tested the power of SOD and each one of these three experts are excited at its potential. Firstly it helps slow down cellular ageing. It does this by neutralising the toxic effects of damaging superoxides that are naturally produced in every cell in your body. If the quantity of superoxides in the cell increases without a corresponding increase in SOD production you have a recipe for accelerated ageing.

A life of exposure to radiation, pollution, drugs and chemical additives found in recreational foods, increases the number of harmful superoxides in and around your cells. This gradual accumulation of superoxides damages the fats, DNA, and overall structure of cells. Take a look at the difference between someone who appears 20 years older than their chronological age, and someone who appears 20 years younger. The difference could be the devastating effect of superoxide free radical damage. SOD seeks out superoxide free radicals and converts them to hydrogen peroxide. Catalase and gluathione peroxide reduce hydrogen peroxide to water before it can combine with another superoxide free radical to form the hydroxyl free radical, the most destructive of all free radicals. It's up to you to use this information to protect yourself because when the supply of SOD is diminished, cells become poisoned and begin to lose their ability to renew themselves, causing premature cellular death. Any abnormal cells in your body are likely to have a greater number of superoxide free radicals within them. SOD occurs naturally in every cell of your body but you can enhance cellular levels by including a daily dose of wheatgrass juice into your routine, it's a superior food source of SOD. Take a look at this study if you're still not convinced.

TESTING THE ELDERLY FOR SOD

Ten senior citizens with an average age of 70 took part in an experiment where they had their blood levels of various nutrients tested before and after taking a wheat sprout supplement. Usually, senior citizens are slower to respond to such experiments, but in this case their serum levels of SOD increased by an average of 230% and by 730% in one individual. 7 out of the 10 more than doubled their blood levels of this powerful antioxidant.

CANCER: OXYGEN DEFICIENCY AT ITS WORSE

Even whilst the struggle against cancer continues, a German biochemist, Dr Otto Warburg, won a Nobel Prize for his research into cancer and oxygen. He discovered that cancer cells thrive in an oxygen-poor environment and concluded that cancer is nothing but a process of cell mutation caused by oxygen deprivation on the cellular level. Even though he arrived at this discovery more than fifty years ago, his theory has never been discredited. Wheatgrass juice contains liquid oxygen that stimulates your digestive system, helps to promote more coherent states of mind and protects against anaerobic bacteria. Start today by eliminating any habit that starves your body of oxygen. Examples are habits such smoking, poor breathing, lack of exercise and diets high in cooked fat.

DESTROY CANCER CELLS WITH B17

There exists another property abundant in wheatgrass juice that selectively destroys cancer cells, leaving non-cancerous ones alone. It was discovered by Dr. Ernst Krebs, Jr. (a highly respected biochemist and researcher) and is known as vitamin B17 (laetrile). In parts of the world where the incidence of cancer is almost non-existent, nutritional intake of vitamin B17 is about 400 times higher than here in the west.

Wheatgrass is also an excellent source of the water-soluble form of vitamin E (atocopherol succinate). It stimulates the production of T-cells, antibodies, interleukin2 and interferon (all factors that enhance immunity) and in this form is very effective in suppressing cancer cell growth. Research with bacteria at the University of Texas Systems Cancer Centre show that chlorophyll may also block the genetic changes that cancer-causing substances produce in cell nuclei. It also has the ability to increase the production of prolactin and growth hormone in the pituitary gland enhancing hormonal balance and control.

STARTING TODAY - A NEW BEGINNING!

Along with wheatgrass juice, eat, blend and juice as many different varieties of raw/wild organic greens as you can! Choose from herbs and big leafy green vegetables. All herbs have rejuvenating properties and some of the more common variety, such as lettuce, celery, parsley, cilantro, etc. are very powerful foods. I blend a lot of spinach and parsley with kale and celery juice. Remember there isn't a laboratory in the world that is a complex as the one found within the photosynthetic green leaf organs of plants.

CHANGE YOUR MOOD, CHANGE YOUR STATE AND GET 'HIGH' ON GREENS!

Did you ever wonder what happens to the body of someone who takes drugs and talks about being 'high'? Have you heard 'drug users' talk about reaching a higher level of being/spirituality when taking drugs? This high is achieved by alkaloids within the drugs alkalising the biochemistry. Although drugs affect the body in many ways, alkaloids have a very specific affect on the body. Essentially alkaloids are bitter organic compounds, derived from plants bearing seeds. Common alkaloids are aspirin, caffeine, cannabinoids (THC, THCV, CBD, CBC), cocaine, morphine, nicotine, etc. If you ever wondered what made hot peppers hot, the answer is alkaloids. Peyote contains the most powerful alkaloids in the world. Look up Peyote on the Internet and you'll see why! The recreational drug Ecstasy, in its original plant form (made from sassafras and nutmeg), contains alkaloids as its active agent.

UNDERSTANDING THE PAIN/PLEASURE PRINCIPLE

When people eat a diet of cooked/processed food and drink highly acidic drinks such as alcohol and cola they develop a very acidic body (a precursor to illness and disease). However, when alkaloids are introduced into the bloodstream via drug use/abuse, they neutralise the acids and allow the user to experience an artificial high as their body and blood is alkalised.

Alkaloids in marijuana smoke neutralise an acidic condition, relax the body, and allow people to feel as if they are tuning into a higher knowledge, a spiritual realm, or connecting with 'something more'. This may sound all well and fine, but there's a physiological price to pay –

the perpetuation of the original problem! Smoking marijuana actually interferes with the ability of the blood to carry sugar, driving carbohydrate cravings through the roof! Many people get high and then experience the so-called 'munchies', hunting out anything that crosses their path (sweets, chocolate, ice-cream, crisps) to restore the body back to its unhealthy acidic condition. The 'higher' you go the more acid-forming foods your body craves to bring you down. If you're smart you'll opt for avocados, nuts, and seeds (acidic raw plant fats) but realistically if you're smoking drugs, your desire for healthy 'raw food' will probably be non-existent. People with the 'munchies' reach for cheese, ice cream, crisps, chocolate and other cooked 'junk' to satisfy such intense cravings!

GO HUNTING FOR WILD GREENS
AND PREPARE FOR THE ULTIMATE 'HIGH'

The idea of eating and juicing more green-leafy vegetables, especially wild herbs, is to significantly alkalise your biochemistry and electrify your blood. Drugs have side effects that can eventually cause serious problems. Greens will just continue to build awesome strength and health. You won't find many alkaloids in fruit, but that shouldn't stop you eating them. Greens should be your primary concern for now. I tend to juice kale, but blend spinach, parsley and other herbs. I also like to add apples or pears to sweeten the juice and make it more palatable. Trust me, when the greens 'kick in', you won't be disappointed! Alkalise your body with greens.

Over time, throw out any coffee/tea, even if you thought you were addicted, and let green juice step in to provide you with (what will feel like) rocket fuel to launch you into your day. If you want to unleash even more raw power into your body and take advantage of a super-food that has four times more chlorophyll than wheatgrass juice, embrace...

E3LIVE - NATURE'S MOST COMPLETE FOOD

Unlike fruits or vegetables that lose many of their vital nutrients during packing and transit, nature has created a food that grows thousands of miles from your door, but can be delivered to you frozen, maintaining every vital nutrient. This food is Aphanizomenon flos-aquae (AFA). It is a blue green algae grown/harvested in its natural state from the mineral rich waters of the Upper Klamath Lake in southern Oregon. It is genetically prepared for extreme alterations in temperature, especially in winter when parts of Klamath Lake freeze over. But when the weather warms up, the algae comes out of its frozen dormancy and resumes its active growth cycle. AFA algae is high in lipids and free fatty acids, which protect it from crystallising in low temperature conditions. Bee pollen works the same way, it can be frozen without losing any of its nutritional value. Marvellous!

WITH FIVE TIMES MORE CHLOROPHYLL THAN WHEATGRASS - ENSURE YOU DON'T MISS OUT!

E3Live has the highest concentration of bio-assimilable chlorophyll than any other food. It has five times more chlorophyll than wheatgrass, twice as much as spirulina algae, and slightly more than chlorella algae. Chlorophyll is the lifeblood of AFA algae and according to biochemist Lita Lee, Ph.D.,

> "Chlorophyll appears to stimulate the regeneration of damaged liver cells, and increases circulation to all organs by dilating blood vessels. In the heart, chlorophyll aids in the transmission of nerve impulses that control contraction. The heart rate is slowed, yet each contraction is increased in power, improving the efficiency of cardiac power."

E3Live is 100% AFA (Aphanizomenon Flos-Aquae). It is 60%+ protein, containing all the amino acids, making it 100% natural brain food. AFA algae is 97% absorbable by the body, contains every B vitamin (including B12) and every known trace mineral. AFA algae contains 10 to 50 times as many minerals as vegetables and is extremely rich in (hard to find) trace minerals, which many people are deficient in. Without trace minerals, enzymatic reactions do not take place within your body. E3Live is also abundant in enzymes, phytochemicals and essential fatty acids, especially the important Omega 3 fatty acids that you need for the formation of eicosanoids. You'll learn about these super-hormones in chapter 8.

DOCTORS ARE PRAISING THIS 'MIRACLE' FOOD

Dr Gabriel Cousins, M.D., holistic physician, psychiatrist and internationally respected author of the classic Conscious Eating has incredible praise for E3Live – "There is no other blue green algae that is alive and active as E3Live. E3Live is the only really live algae we have now. The life force aspect of E3Live is probably the most important factor that singles it out. E3Live has the strongest possible effects, and represents a qualitative leap compared to any other algae coming out of Klamath Lake"

E3LIVE AND ATHLETIC PEAK PERFORMANCE

Many athletes have broken through their limits and gone on to achieve remarkable success in their chosen field by choosing E3Live as one of their preferred forms of nutrition. Do you want to join this elite group, who are smashing personal bests and becoming champions in their chosen endeavour? Here are just a few:

- Grant Hackett, Long Distance Swimmer, 2000 Olympic Gold Medal Winner in the 1500 meter freestyle.
- Ky Hurst – Australian Iron man Triathlete Champion.
- Mary Louise Zeller – 57 year old Tae Kwon Do US National Champion, Gold Medal International Champion competing against opponents 40 years younger.
- Lynne Taylor – Miss Natural Olympia 1999 – Drug-free World Champion Body-Builder – Mother of Four.
- Ryk Neethling – Olympic Swimmer and World Record Holder.

HORMONAL CONTROL AND BRAIN REGULATION – NORMALISE BLOOD SUGAR LEVELS WITH E3LIVE

E3 Live is a valuable asset to anyone suffering with diabetes. The elements within it assist in the restoration of an over-worked pancreas. With its exceptional blood sugar balancing qualities, it helps eliminate the craving for alcohol and drugs whilst enhancing brain function (brain function is immediately optimised when blood sugar levels are stabilised.) You'll learn more about the importance of keeping your blood sugar levels optimised in chapter 11.

EXPEL PROZAC FROM THE EARTH –
USE E3LIVE TO RESTORE MENTAL HEALTH

E3Live is incredibly rich in amino acids, providing the necessary raw materials for the brain to manufacture serotonin-based neuro-transmitters. These go on to support the master glands of the entire endocrine system, creating a harmonious inner environment. You'll discover the power of neurotransmitters in chapter 14.

RESTORING BRAIN FUNCTION AND BALANCE
TO YOUR CENTRAL NERVOUS SYSTEM

The brains of drug addicts and alcoholics are often functioning very poorly. They have unbalanced brain wave readings, and a lack of mood and memory control. By using E3Live along with other dietary changes, electroencephalogram (EEG) readings can be normalised, if not optimised, restoring balance to the central nervous system.

As long as someone's brain function is only 'sub-clinically' out of balance showing unbalanced EEG readings (and not dramatically out of balance like those who suffer epileptic seizures), E3Live can help to restore balance and harmony. There isn't a supplemental food as pure and natural as the AFA algae found in E3Live.

BOLSTERING UP YOUR IMMUNE SYSTEM WITH E3LIVE

A recent study showed that E3Live activates up to 40% more of the immune system's beneficial natural killer cells. These cells hunt out viruses and bacteria, even if they are deep within the body's tissues. According to Dr Gabriel Cousins, AFA algae has some anti-HIV effects, although more research needs to be done in these areas.

POWER UP YOUR VITAMIN B12 STATUS
AND MAXIMISE YOUR OXYGEN UPTAKE

AFA has the highest active vegetable source of vitamin B12, in a form that is totally usable by the body. It has 65 times more B12 than kelp and 700 times more B12 than alfalfa. Without enough vitamin B12 oxygen uptake is compromised and according to Dr. Otto Warburg, oxygen deprivation is the major cause of cancer.

The key difference between taking supplements and taking E3Live is that the AFA algae found in E3Live is recognised by the body as food. This means it is immediately available with a greater than 90% assimilation rate. It is so powerful, NASA have been studying the algae as a possible food source for space missions and Russians have used it to treat patients exposed to radiation in the Chernobyl nuclear disaster.

MAINTAINING THE CRITICAL
ACID/ALKALINE BALANCE IN YOUR BODY

Green leafy vegetables in your diet counteract the acid forming nature of raw plant fats such as nuts, seeds and avocados. Many vegetarians/vegans eat a lot of fruit. Fruits contain slightly more phosphorus than calcium so end up being more acidic in their final breakdown. Without enough alkalising greens in your diet your body will take on more of an acidic nature. Green leafy vegetables provide the necessary alkalinity to prolong exceptional health and allow you to maintain an excellent calcium-phosphorus balance. More about balancing raw foods in chapter 8.

By consuming at least 2.5 pounds of (1.1kg) of green leafed vegetables daily (1/3 eaten, 2/3 juiced) you'll rebuild stores of the critical minerals calcium, magnesium, and silicon.

The best green leafed vegetables include:

Bok choy, celery (very important, an excellent source of sodium), cilantro, crane's bill, collard, dandelion, dark green cabbage, endive, fennel (wild), kale (especially dinosaur kale), lamb's quarters (goose foot), lettuce (all types), malva, mustard (wild), parsley, spinach, spring onions (green), sunflower greens, wild radish, all green herbs, all wild edible greens, algae (blue-green, chlorella, and spirulina, these are alkaline green protein foods, they are not true leafy-vegetables, but can be used in this category).

Nature's Living Superfood is another excellent addition to your diet and can be ordered along with E3 Live Blue-Green Algae from the Fresh Network 0870 800 7070 www.fresh-network.com or Kiki Health 01493 857878 www.kiki-health.com. Outside of the UK you can contact www.rawfood.com.

ARE YOU READY FOR THE CHALLENGE?

The most important part of RAW PERFECTION is building the foundation for success. First you make your positive addictions and then you tackle your negative ones. Throughout our journey together you'll discover what the best foods to eat are and why. You'll learn to work with them, play with them and experiment like never before until you discover what tickles your taste buds.

In the absence of light there's darkness, and these early principles shine the light of nutritional success down upon you. Look to the light and you won't see the shadows. Look to the light and your old negative addictions will fade away and be forgotten!

Wheatgrass juice, E3Live or any raw green juice should be the first thing you drink when you wake in the morning, and the last thing you drink at night. You'll feel it rushing through your body every time you drink it, raising the hair on the back of your neck. Here's a re-cap why:

- ◆ Numerous experiments on animal and human subjects have shown chlorophyll to be effective in treating anaemia (a low serum iron count).
- ◆ Wheatgrass juice and E3Live contain every amino acid necessary for a life of vitality. These amino acid chains (polypeptides), are absorbed directly into your blood, and can neutralise toxic substances like cadmium, nicotine, strontium, mercury, and polyvinyl chloride, by changing them into insoluble salts that your body can eliminate more easily.
- ◆ Wheatgrass juice and E3Live are both rapidly assimilated by your body and help stimulate cellular metabolism.
- ◆ Wheatgrass and E3Live are rich supplies of bioflavinoids and used to help cleanse the blood and tissues, detoxifying cells and preventing their deterioration.
- ◆ Wheatgrass juice and E3Live will cause your blood vessels to dilate, leading to an increase in overall blood flow. The delivery of nutrients to your cells will be enhanced, the elimination of waste speeded up and with an increased blood flow, oxygen delivery is enhanced.
- ◆ Choline, magnesium and potassium are three compounds found abundantly in wheatgrass. They are essential for detoxification and help the liver stay vital and healthy.
- ◆ Even offensive body odour can be neutralised if chlorophyll is consumed consistently over the course of a few weeks.

- Wheatgrass is an abundant source of enzymes, which among other things help to detoxify the pollutants that are part of every day life. They also increase your ability to digest food more fully, dissolve excesses of fat and protein, and in some cases may even break down tumours and cysts.

- Wheatgrass is a superior food source of Superoxide dimutase (SOD), the true anti-ageing enzyme.

- P4D1 and D1G1 are two glyco-proteins found in wheatgrass that have excellent anti-inflammatory actions, anti-ulcer actions and a powerful antioxidant potential. P4D1 has the ability to stimulate the production and natural repair of human reproductive sperm cells and DNA.

- Wheatgrass is abundant in vitamin B17 (laetrile) which can selectively destroy cancer cells, leaving non-cancerous ones alone.

- Wheatgrass has the power to simultaneously neutralise the toxic effect of fluorine, and convert it into an ally that helps in the maintenance of healthy bones and teeth.

- 2oz of wheatgrass juice has the equivalent vitamin and mineral content of roughly 4lbs of organic green vegetables. On an empty stomach, it is assimilated into the blood in about 20 minutes and is charged with 'chi' electrical energy. The vitality lasts throughout the day.

- Wheatgrass juice has been shown to build red blood cells quickly after ingestion. It normalises high blood pressure and stimulates healthy tissue-cell growth.

- Drs Hugh and Latner found that small doses of **pure** chlorophyll regenerate blood haemoglobin levels, but large doses appeared to be toxic to bone marrow. **Crude** chlorophyll, on the other hand was found to be non toxic even in large doses.

- Chlorophyll doesn't play much of a role in medicine because its inherent instability prevents it from being stored. Like fresh fats and oils, fresh vegetable and fruit juice, when exposed to light and air deteriorate/oxidise very rapidly.

- If you have any concerns about osteoporosis, let them be banished. Chlorophyll promotes calcium absorption because it has a similar action to vitamin D in your body. When you consume wheatgrass juice, you'll also be tapping into an excellent source of vitamins A and C and the mineral magnesium, all of which help you absorb more calcium.

- Grass juice and E3Live are excellent transition and detoxification foods (especially for overcoming heavy metal poisoning). The earth is covered with grass. Four of the world's top five crops come from it.

Muscular 2000lb animals sustain themselves on it and science has found every nutrient in it.

♦ Having spent many years researching plant foods, Brian Clement, director of Hippocrates Health Institute in West Palm Beach, Florida, has reported that wild greens have the highest energy frequency of any food. Wild greens should be your preference, but if you can't get wild you should buy organic!

♦ Anyone who attempts to sell you on the idea of becoming vegan or vegetarian better also sell you on the idea of drinking raw wheatgrass juice/raw greens, blue green algae, sprouts and raw plant fats. Without them, it can be easier to form addictions to foods that over-stimulate the hormone insulin, and lead you down a path towards an early grave. Many vegetarians are addicted to pasta, bread, cheese and rice. See chapter 8 and 9 for more information

Greens balance the acid-forming minerals (sulphur, chloride, and phosphorus) found in avocados, nuts, seeds, onions, garlic, etc. (all of which are critical on an all-raw diet). No one food should be eaten exclusively, but greens should definitely form the foundation on which you want to build true balance! Not only do they deliver an abundance of nutrients and vitality, but they'll also cause you to feel very centred!

The choice is yours – dead food and a lifeless body – or live raw food and a vibrant body. As Dr. Bernard Jensen said, "If you're green on the inside, you're clean on the inside."

THE RAW PERFECTION EVALUATION:
Do you juice up to 4oz of wheatgrass daily?
Have you begun to use E3live on a daily basis?
Do you create a variety of green drinks that tickle your taste buds?

The germinating seed represents a protein-manufacturing machine, which is turning out protein...along with necessary vitamins and minerals for its assimilation and utilisation
- Dr.Jeffrey Bland, Biochemist, University of Puget Sound

CHAPTER 3

HARNESSING THE MIRACLE OF NATURE: SPROUT POWER

In the 1970s, Loretta Harmony Kohn underwent medical treatment for a variety of difficulties. The most problematical were two brain seizures. Shortly after the treatment she was diagnosed with epilepsy and her driving licence revoked. Her physical condition deteriorated and as time drifted by she suffered with severe depression. In 1979, after her second epileptic seizure, she felt alone, stranded and wanted to give up on life. On the brink of suicide she read a book by the late Ann Wigmore entitled, 'Be Your Own Doctor: Let Living food Be Your Medicine'. Ann's approach was to use raw foods for healing, none more important than sprouted alfalfa seeds, wheat berry sprouts and wheatgrass juice.

INSPIRATION LEAD TO REGENERATION

Having been inspired by what she had read, Loretta made the decision to visit The Hippocrates Health Institute in Boston, Massachusetts, founded by Ann. She packed her belongings and moved there for one month in a last ditch effort to regain her health.

Ann informed Loretta that her seizures were due to an over toxic body. Years of nutritional/lifestyle abuse had got her into this mess, but raw plant foods were going to help her out of it! When Ann was alive she worked with hundreds of sick people, relying on 'live foods' (sprouted salads, sprouted juices, and other sprouted foods) to eject, eradicate and expel the toxic sludge from their bodies. People often arrived barely able to move or speak, and left being able to walk, run, swim and play tennis!

SIMPLE RITUALS, POWERFUL RESULTS

As part of Loretta's routine she was given juice in the morning made with 50% alfalfa and 50% wheat sprouts, a salad or sandwich abundant in alfalfa and wheat sprouts for lunch, and another sprout juice with a baked vegetarian sprout loaf or vegetable/sprout burgers for dinner. Within a few short days, excess fat began melting off her body and her energy began to replenish. For 120 days she continued these simple rituals until she felt convinced she was healed. At this point she wanted medical proof. She decided to visit a physician at Brigham and Women's Hospital in Boston and submitted herself to have an electroencephalogram (EEG). When the results came back from the laboratory, Loretta couldn't believe it! The liberating diet Ann had given her had not only allowed her to recover from her low energy and depression, but had also freed her from epileptic seizures. Loretta could begin driving again.

CREATING A MAGICAL DIET FROM MAGICAL MATERIALS

One of the mysteries that has puzzled scientists for years is how one tiny seed can develop into a fully grown plant. With this in mind it is time to embrace the power of sprouted seeds, grains, nuts and pulses.

- The pulses: Peanuts, adzuki beans, chickpeas, lima beans, blackeye peas, soybeans, kidney beans, lentils, mung beans, navy beans, etc.
- The Seeds: Pumpkin, sunflower, mustard, fenugreek, alfalfa, radish, buckwheat, sesame, etc.
- The Nuts: Brazil nuts, almonds, hazelnuts, pine nuts, pecans, pistachios, walnuts, cashews, etc.
- The Grains: Quinoa, rye, rice, oats, millet, wheat, barley, maize, etc.

In their original form, these foods have a very low water content and are very concentrated. However, when they are sprouted their nutritional content rises dramatically. Sprouts are alive and are capable of transferring their life-force to you! They represent the most natural, healthiest foods in existence. They cost next to nothing to produce and will supply you with...

PERFECT NUTRITION AND PERFECT HEALTH

You've seen how a tiny seed can sprout and force it's way through a slab of stone! Well imagine what that kind of life-force and energy can do for you! Each and every seed contains enough stored energy to send it on its way in life, and all the genetic information necessary to grow and develop into a plant. These intelligent little powerhouses know up from down, light from dark and moist from dry.

Pound for pound, sprouted pulses, seeds, nuts and grains are more nutritious, cheaper and fresher than any other food. They are probably the most underestimated food available in society today. Very little expenditure or effort is needed to grow them and they will improve your diet beyond comprehension.

Sprouts deliver a number of life-enhancing benefits, making them nutritional super-foods:

♦ They represent the freshest food you can eat, as they grow energetically right up until the moment they are eaten.
♦ Pound for pound they are the cheapest food in existence with a higher nutrient ratio than any other food.
♦ You can eat them raw, which makes them a quick and easy food for a busy lifestyle.
♦ Because they are eaten raw, all vital elements are kept intact.
♦ You can grow them in your own home and have total control over their production. Sprouts are a very clean, safe food to eat.
♦ They are rich in natural plant enzymes that must to be present in your diet if you ever want to maximise the efficiency of your digestive system.

SPROUTS, UNLIMITED HEALTH AND
CANCER PREVENTION?

As far back as 1978 Dr. Charles Shaw and Dr. Chiu-Nan at the University of Texas Cancer Centre tested a variety of foods to determine whether they had any anti-cancer properties. The chosen foods included lentil sprouts, mung bean sprouts, wheat sprouts, as well as carrots and parsley. The foods were then tested on mice inoculated with carcinogens (cancer causing substances). Although the carrots and parsley did show an inhibitory effect on the carcinogens, the true heroes of the experiment were the sprouts. They inhibited the activity of the carcinogens, even when small dosages of the sprout extracts were used. The other major benefit was that the extract wasn't toxic even in high dosages. (Most known inhibitors of carcinogens are toxic at even moderately high levels of concentration.) With this information fresh in your mind, let me introduce you to...

THE POWER OF SPROUTED BEANS

Sprouted beans represent a truly magical form of nutrition, not only do they provide an abundance of hunger-cutting protein, but they also replace the calcium that is lost through diets high in animal protein.

- ◆ Let over-nutrition satiate you – Sprouted beans are so nutritionally dense and high in fibre, your body will feel very satisfied after eating only a small quantity. Their bulkiness and low-calorie make-up make them the perfect food for life-extension. (Calorie restriction is the only proven method of increasing longevity. More about this later.)
- ◆ Improve your blood profile – Long-term studies carried out by Dr. James W. Anderson at the University of Kentucky showed that as little as 50grams of beans per day can reduce serum cholesterol levels and actually increase serum HDL-cholesterol levels. Avoid cooking beans if you can sprout them. By doing so you'll preserve the vital nutrients that assist in their digestion and assimilation.
- ◆ Keep blood glucose levels balanced – The soluble fibre in sprouted beans gels in the intestines and prevents any dramatic rises in blood sugar, the importance of this will become apparent in later chapters. For now, remember that stable blood sugar levels are synonymous with awesome energy levels and peak performance states of mind.

♦ Sprouted beans energise – Beans contain high levels of the amino acid tyrosine. You'll read about tyrosine in chapter 14 – Food For Thought. It is a critical amino-acid necessary for the synthesis of the neurotransmitter dopamine. As you spark the fire of your brain's dopamine receptors, your outlook on the world will become more positive. You'll feel more energy and vigour, cut stress and develop laser-like concentration, all whilst feeling more lively and buoyant. Dopamine also increases your sexual vigour and helps you to exercise longer.

♦ Sprout and be free from the wind – It was discovered at the U.S. Department of Agriculture near Berkeley, California that a group of complex sugars called oligo saccharides found in beans cause excessive flatulence. Fortunately though, when a bean is sprouted it secretes an enzyme called glastosidase. This enzyme breaks down the sugars and prevents the formation of excessive gas.

21ST CENTURY SUPER FOOD
IN ANY SEASON FOR ANY REASON

If your finances became tight, you could live healthily and well on 30p of sprouts a day. Sprouted seeds and grains can be grown in any season of the year, regardless of the weather conditions or climate. They are also quick to harvest, just lift them from the seed tray, rinse them and store them in your refrigerator until they are needed. Growing them at home takes no time at all! You will have a new harvest every few days.

IGNITING THE FLAME OF YOUR SEXUAL FIRE
WITH SEXY SPROUTS

One interesting study performed by the Agricultural Experiment Station in Beltsville, Maryland demonstrated the ability of sprouted grains to restore fertility to cows that lost or outgrew their ability to reproduce. One study used cows that had never shown any signs of reproductive capacity. Each animal was fed five pounds of sprouted oats daily along with its usual food. Would you believe that after just sixty days all the cows were pregnant!

I don't know how you assess your sexual vigour, but since Viagra 'popped up' a few years ago, it has become one of the fastest selling prescription drugs in history. I'll let you make you mind up about how seriously people take their sexual prowess. Let sprouts be your starting point if you need your sexual functions rejuvenated and restored to their normal healthy state.

Sprouted seeds are an important part of the diet of the long-lived Hunza people of the Himalayas and if you want to know more about this group of people, wait until you get to the end of this book. You'll learn that not only does their culture have one of the highest percentages of centenarians, but they are also very active up until the time they pass away, especially sexually! They also have very efficient digestive systems, which brings me onto the subject of enzyme inhibitors...

DESTROYING ENZYME INHIBITORS
COOKING -V- SPROUTING

Seeds need to be tough to survive the most adverse of conditions and all the nutrients within them are packed away in a tough woody matrix. Normally we'd cook beans and pulses to soften this matrix, destroying the unfavourable enzyme inhibitors. The only problem here is that cooking also destroys the beneficial plant enzymes that you require to make the food complete. If the essential plant enzymes are destroyed, your body will have to release extra enzymes from the pancreas to make up the difference, thus taxing your system. Many people in Western civilisation have an enlarged and overworked pancreas because they put such great demands on their pancreas by eating so much cooked food. In fact, compared to any other species on earth, in proportion to body size and weight, humans have the largest pancreas in existence.

♦ Chickpeas contain a substance called a trypsin inhibitor. This substance blocks the action of some of the enzymes in the body which break down protein, leaving some of the valuable amino acids useless and unavailable to the body. Trypsin in chickpeas is rendered harmless by sprouting, but not by cooking.

♦ Soybeans, broad beans and red kidney beans also contain a trypsin inhibitor. Researchers have discovered that soybeans will not support life unless they are cooked for several hours. Cooking neutralises the trypsin inhibitor, but at the expense of also killing many of the nutrients that make soybeans such a powerful food. Sprouting does the same job whilst ensuring the beans maintain all of their powerful nutritional make-up. Ensure that when you soak them, you change the water every 4-8 hours.

FIGHTING AGAINST PHYTIN
WITH THE POWER OF SPROUTING

Your body can only assimilate minerals properly if they are part of organic molecules. Vegetable foods are an excellent source of organic minerals, but in foods such as peas, beans and some grains there are substances that bind with minerals to form insoluble compounds that the body can't deal with. Phytic acid is one of these substances and it binds with iron, calcium and zinc preventing their absorption. Phytin is a magnesium-calcium salt of phytic acid and is also found in the makeup of many seeds. Like phytic acid it is rich in phosphorus and can represent as much as 80% of the phosphorus content of some seeds. When you begin sprouting you dramatically decrease the content of these undesirable phosphates (such as phytin), transforming a potentially hazardous food into a complete super-food!

In the process of germination, as well as an increase in vitamin and mineral content, the desirable phosphorus compounds such as lecithin also increase. You'll learn later how lecithin is critical in:

♦ Optimising mental performance and brain power.
♦ Maintaining a healthy nervous system.
♦ Breaking up and transporting fats and fatty acids around the body.
♦ Preventing too many acids or alkaline substances accumulating in the blood.
♦ Stimulating the secretion of hormones and encouraging the transport of nutrients though cell walls.
♦ Maintaining efficient fat metabolism.

THE POWER OF PRAYER... SOMETHING TO THINK ABOUT

A botanist by the name of Dr Robert Jerome, at the University of Mexico, found that by intentionally sending out loving thoughts to his plants, he was able to make them grow much faster. He also discovered that by sending out hateful thoughts, he was able to cause plants to wither and die in five weeks (even when receiving proper care of soil, water and sunlight). It makes you wonder doesn't it? Prayed over seeds grow faster than ones that are left to their own devices. Minister Franklin Loehr and his researchers have performed experiments with 20,000 seeds and have satisfactorily demonstrated that prayer affects germination and growth if it is done repeatedly.

SPROUTED SOYBEANS: THE WONDER FOOD

Clive McCay, professor of nutrition at Cornell University, once researched the sprouted soybean and declared that he had discovered an almost perfect food.

♦ It will grow in any climate.
♦ It rivals meat in nutritional value.
♦ It matures in 3-5 days whatever time of year it is planted.
♦ It requires neither soil nor sunshine.
♦ It rivals tomatoes in vitamin C.
♦ It is free of waste in preparation.

Soybeans supply almost all of the essential amino acids, have more protein than any other bean and supply an abundance of omega 3 fatty acids.

Soy isoflavones are the active ingredient in soybeans, and are known to inhibit a number of adverse reactions, acting as powerful antioxidants. Genistein, a major soy isoflavone, inhibits the growth of a number of cancer cells in laboratory tests and inhibits blood vessel growth essential for tumour cell growth. This is one of the reasons why soy is so powerful in preventing Breast and Prostate cancer.

The list of benefits associated with soybeans is almost endless. They have double the dietary fibre of wheat and double the protein content of many meats. Soy isoflavones reduce the risk of osteoporosis and should be considered vital by vegetarians, which brings me to an important point. I've often found the mentality of vegetarians to be less than useful in their quest for health. They only focus on cutting out meats, without saturating their diet with an abundance of quality foods that ensure they have unlimited health. It's not as easy to control various hormones without the use of meat, unless you include sprouts in your diet. Without sprouts, it won't be as easy for you to supply the essential nutrients vital for RAW PERFECTION. Studies show that vegetarian women who have high intakes of soy protein have lower rates of osteoporosis. Soybeans have a very low glycemic index of 15. They cause minimal fluctuations in blood sugar levels making them a perfect food for weight loss and for controlling problems such as diabetes. Begin eating more of them today and you'll...

BEGIN THE JOURNEY TOWARDS
A PEAK PERFORMANCE MIND

In the final section when you've really begun to master the principles of RAW PERFECTION, you'll learn more about acetylcholine. It is the most abundant neurotransmitter in the brain and essential to higher mental processes such as learning and memory. If you want to improve your learning ability and intelligence, whilst developing a mind that can concentrate like a laser, ensure you maintain high levels of this neurotransmitter in your brain. If you don't you will almost certainly suffer from memory loss and cognitive dysfunction. The answer: Eat more soy products, especially sprouted soybeans. The precursor for acetylcholine is choline and soy is a very rich source. If you are an athlete...

USE SOY TO PREVENT THE PHYSIOLOGICAL
HAZARDS OF ENDURANCE EVENTS

When the blood profiles of marathon runners were studied, choline levels fluctuated dramatically. Researcher Richard Wurtman discovered that after 26 miles of running, choline drops by a staggering 40%. Studies also show that swimmers are able to swim for longer (without the perils of muscle fatigue) when choline is introduced into their diet. Eat sprouted soybeans and you'll be one step closer to mastery.

NEVER EAT NUTS OR SEEDS RAW
IF YOU CAN SPROUT THEM

In an experiment in 1944, young rats and chickens were fed a diet of raw soybeans (high in enzyme inhibitors). In order to combat the enzyme inhibitors, huge quantities of pancreatic digestive enzymes were produced to assist digestion, and as expected the pancreas of animals gradually enlarged, causing stunted growth and sickness. Ensure you soak soybeans for at least 24 hours prior to sprouting them and change the soak water every 4-8 hours. The message: Soak your nuts and seeds and turn them into sprouts!

ALFALFA SPROUTS – THE BASIS OF QUALITY NUTRITION

Alfalfa sprouts are possibly one of the most nutritionally rich foods you'll ever eat. Not only do they have an amazingly high vitamin and mineral content, but they contain every amino acid, with a protein content around 40%. Add to this the anti-toxin properties that surpass those of liver, brewer's yeast and wheat germ, and you can easily see why they are so essential to your diet. People have eaten alfalfa sprouts and experienced remission from a number of ailments. They provide an excellent calcium-phosphorus ratio (2:1). They supply your body with a large quantity of low-calorie liquid nourishment that is easily digested and used as fuel. In addition, the liquid helps to flush toxins out of the body and is an excellent source of trace elements such as iodine, zinc, selenium, chromium, cobalt, and silicon. Alfalfa sprouts and sprouted pumpkin seeds are especially potent sources of zinc. Zinc is necessary for the synthesis of protein, liver functions, and the healing of cuts and wounds. Selenium is abundant in alfalfa sprouts and is now being tested for anti-cancer properties.

GANGRENE CURED WITH ALFALFA SPROUT JUICE

In the late 1970s, a middle aged man suffering from gangrene in his right leg visited Ann Wigmore at her institute. Poor circulation due to acute diabetes had been the cause of this problem, but Ann seemed to have the answer. She gave him four glasses of alfalfa and wheat sprout juice to drink daily. To make this juice, simply put equal parts with a little water in a blender for three minutes. Ann also used the concoction for bathing the afflicted limb on a daily basis. Can you believe it took only two weeks for the gangrene to completely heal!

MUNG BEAN SPROUTS –
THE MAGICAL SPROUT/FRUIT LINK

Fruit has the power to cleanse your body, heal you and provide you with unlimited energy. The interesting link between mung bean sprouts and fruit is that after 5 days of sprouting, apart from appearance, they virtually match each others nutritional content. Mung beans sprouts have a carbohydrate content virtually identical to that found in a casaba melon. They increase in water content from 10.7% found in the seed to 88.8% in the sprout. The protein content is similar to that found in a dry fig, whilst its calorie content is similar to that of a papaya or honeydew melon. Mung sprouts have a vitamin C content similar to that found in a pineapple, vitamin A content of a lemon, thiamine content of an avocado, riboflavin content of an apple, niacin content of a banana, calcium content of damson plums, potassium level of papaya and iron percentage of a loganberry. Mung bean sprouts also rival soybeans sprouts in health benefits. The isoflavones and phytoestrogens are known to prevent disease, whilst creating beneficial bacteria in your gastrointestinal tract. Mung sprouts are good sources of the iron needed for red blood cell formation and the transport of oxygen from the lungs to the cells. You've discovered the power of alfalfa sprouts and mung beans. Now it's time for you to...

GO NUTS ABOUT NUTS!

In the next chapter I will introduce you to the power of raw plant fats. For now, I would like to point out that without out the essential omega 3 fatty acids, your health could be in danger! A great way to get extra omega 3s in your diet is to go a little nuts for nuts! Researchers recently found that women who ate nuts regularly had a 32% lower risk of having a non-fatal heart attack and were 39% less likely to die of a heart attack than those who never or rarely consumed nuts. The amount of nuts needed to provide the protection was very low – only five ounces a week. A handful of walnuts, macadamias, almonds, pecans, or hazelnuts can do more for your health than you think. Similar results from the Physician's Health Study suggest that frequent nut consumption benefit men in the same way.

BRAZIL NUTS FIGHT THE CANCER BATTLE

Brazil nuts have been found to increase cancer resistance due to their exceptionally high levels of selenium. Researchers at Roswell Park Cancer Institute showed that animals fed the tropical nut increased their resistance to tumours more significantly than a group fed a walnut-enriched diet. Even supplementation of selenium didn't prove any more powerful than eating a daily serving of brazil nuts. When it comes to the anti-cancer properties of selenium, brazil nuts lead the pack.

TAKE MACADAMIA NUTS TO HEART

Macadamia nuts have been found to improve fat metabolism efficiency according to a preliminary study conducted by researchers at the University of Hawaii in Honolulu. High levels of omega 6 fatty acids counteract the beneficial effects of omega 3 fatty acids. Macadamia oil has only 3% omega 6 fatty acids.

POWERFUL PISTACHIOS PACK A MIND BOOSTING PUNCH

In a study back in the 1960s, alcoholics were given the opportunity to relieve their addiction by taking part in an experiment using high doses of glutamic acid (GA). They were given 2 grams, 3 times a day for the first month, 12 grams a day for the second month and finally 15 grams for month 3 and 4. Compared to the control group taking placebos, 75% of the experimental group reported remarkable control over their drinking habits. By deciding to eat a cup of pistachios every day, you'll be ingesting about 6 grams of GA. Pistachios are excellent at supplying you energy as well. Glutamic acid forms a partnership with gamma-aminobutyric acid (GABA) and glutamine (GAM) causing your brain reactions to run more smoothly. GA is a stimulating neurotransmitter, whilst GABA calms the brain. GAM on the other hand performs so many different functions it's hard to classify. Out of all the amino acids, GA is the most abundant one in the brain and its main role is to help in the production of mental energy. If you're doing anything that requires intense mental concentration and an excellent memory, and you want a snack, choose a cup of shelled pistachios.

USING WALNUTS IN THE FIGHT AGAINST HEART DISEASE

In the spring of 1993 researchers at Loma Linda University Medical School (California) made some exciting discoveries. They reported that after comparing the results of two four week long dietary intervention trials in 18 men, eating moderate amounts of walnuts, without increasing total dietary fat and calories, "decreases serum cholesterol levels and favourably modifies the lipoprotein profile in healthy men."

LOAD UP YOUR DIET WITH ANTIOXIDANT FOODS

The amino acids cysteine and glutathione are powerful antioxidants. They protect against car exhaust fumes, carcinogens, infections, alcohol excess and toxic metals. They also help make one of the body's key antioxidant enzymes, and help detoxify the body. Cysteine and glutathione are particularly high in lentils, beans, nuts, seeds, onions and garlic. They have been shown to boost the immune system and increase antioxidant power.

POWER UP YOUR ANTIOXIDANT STATUS
WITH ELLAGIC ACID

In the October 1968 Journal of Pharmaceutical Sciences (57:1730-31) you can read a study where ellagic acid from black walnuts was injected into a group of mice before they underwent electroconvulsive shock. With the presence of this substance in their blood they remained alive for longer than other rodents that were shocked but received no injections. This suggests that ellagic acid has a protective effect on the myelin sheathing (fatty protein substance) encasing each strand of nerve.

Between 1985 and 1990 researchers at the Medical College of Ohio in Toledo began investigating ellagic acids effects on cancer growth. They found that ellagic acid competes for DNA receptors that are also used by carcinogens. Thus with more ellagic acid in your diet you give your body greater strength and a greater chance against the diseases of modern civilisation. Ellagic acid is found in blackcurrants, grapes, raspberries, strawberries, and some nuts such as brazil nuts and walnuts.

RAW PERFECTION RITUAL:
THE SESAME, SUNFLOWER, PUMPKIN SEED MIX

Seeds such as sunflower, pumpkin and sesame seeds are excellent sources of protein, essential fatty acids, vitamins, minerals and trace elements. They are rich in magnesium and calcium. The minerals in sprouts are chelated; that is, in their natural state, they are chemically bound to amino acids, so that the human body easily assimilates them.

If you sprout an equal quantity of sunflower, pumpkin and sesame seeds and blend them in a drink with a banana, some Tahini and some soaked almonds you'll have a very powerful nutrient rich drink that will serve your body and unleash awesome health! Take a look for yourself:

Sprout	Nutritional Make-up
Sesame	Calcium, magnesium, phosphorous, vitamins B and E plus essential fatty acids.
Sunflower	Vitamins A, C, minerals and chlorophyll.
Pumpkin	Vitamin E, amino acids, essential fatty acids, B vitamins, phosphorous, iron and zinc.
Almond	Alkaline protein, vitamins B & E plus unsaturated fatty acids, rich source of calcium.

ARE YOU READY FOR THE CHALLENGE?

The Power of sprouts is second to none. They can be used as a weapon against disease and illness and help secure good health when combined with the other principles of RAW PERFECTION. If you see sprouting as a problem there is only one solution: Go out and buy one packet of as many different varieties of nuts, seeds, pulses and grains, and make it your commitment to sprout all of them. Treat it like your ultimate experiment. Call it personal responsibility. It represents the beginning of a richer, more fulfilling life. Be the best you've ever been. Now is the time and sprouts are your tool to turn your dreams of health into reality. They are the all-singing, all-dancing super food that will propel you down the road towards scintillating health. Here's a re-cap:

♦ Sprouts are low on the glycemic index and help keep blood sugar balanced. This is critical for consistent energy and optimal brain function.

♦ Sprouts offer all the nutrients essential for maximum vitality. Levels of vitamins and minerals increase during the sprouting process. Some as high as 600%.

♦ Sprouted beans supply high levels of the amino acid tyrosine, a critical building block for dopamine – the neurotransmitter that affects how alert you are.

♦ Sprouts form part of the diet of the long-lived Hunza people of the Himalayas. They have one of the highest percentages of centenarians in existence today.

- Sprouts increase the micro-electrical potential of cells, improving your body's use of oxygen so that both muscles and brain are energised.

- In the process of germination the desirable phosphorus compounds such as lecithin increase.

- Sprouted beans provide an abundance of hunger-cutting protein and replace the calcium that is lost through diets high in animal protein. They fill you up, improve your blood profile, keep blood glucose levels balanced and energise you.

- Sprouted soybeans grow in any climate, rival meat in nutritional value, mature within 3-5 days of sprouting, require neither soil nor sunshine, rival tomatoes in vitamin C and are full of soy isoflavones, known to inhibit growth of cancer cells in laboratory tests.

- Alfalfa sprouts provide an excellent calcium-phosphorus ratio (2:1) and are excellent sources of trace elements such as iodine, zinc, selenium, chromium, cobalt and silicon.

- Mung bean sprouts also rival soybean sprouts. The isoflavones and phytoestrogens are known to prevent disease, whilst creating beneficial bacteria in your gastrointestinal tract.

- Brazil nuts pack a healthy selenium punch offering anti-cancer properties. Macadamia nuts have been found to improve fat metabolism. Pistachio nuts are excellent brain food, and walnuts help develop optimal blood profiles.

- Remember to pray for your sprouts and watch as your loving thoughts cause them to grow full of life and vitality.

THE RAW PERFECTION EVALUATION:
Do you sprout your own pulses, seeds, nuts or grains?
Do you eat them on a regular basis?
Do you drink the powerful sesame, sunflower, pumpkin, almond sprout drink?

CHAPTER 4

THE POWER OF RAW PLANT FATS

In Europe, before the Second World War, oil pressing was a home and cottage industry. Every large estate and small town usually had an oil mill and many villages had an oil beater.

The oil beater would put flax or other seeds into a funnel, place a steel wedge on top of the seeds, and then pound the wedge with a sledge hammer – crushing the seeds and pressing the oil into a barrel. Once or twice a week the oil beater would put the barrel of oil onto his wagon and ride through the village selling it. People stored the fresh pressed oil in a ceramic container in a cool dark place. Storage was critical because of its short shelf life. It was treated like milk, eggs and bread, spoiling quickly if not consumed.

In the 1920s the oil trade became big business and almost over night people discovered how to press oils in huge quantities and preserve them for greater profit. Unfortunately the oils produced (like the ones on the supermarket shelves today) were chemically refined for more stability and longer shelf life, pale in colour, and bland in taste, most lacking the essential fatty acids, linoleic acid (an omega 6 fatty acid) and linolenic acid (an omega 3 fatty acid).

HIGH FAT, LOW FAT OR NO FAT - WHAT'S THE STORY?

People have been conditioned to think that all fat is bad. This is only a half-truth. Raw plant fats are in fact one of the most important nutrients you could possibly eat, along with green leafy vegetation, fruits, vegetables and sprouts.

WHY ALL THE FUSS ABOUT FAT?

Simple. The majority of fat eaten in Western civilisation is cooked. Cooked fat kills! Whenever fat is cooked, trans-fatty acids are produced, and they represent one of the most destructive elements of any cooked food diet. Here's why:

◆ They are a major source of damaging free radicals.
◆ They are very difficult to digest without their associated enzyme lipase.
◆ They strip you of your energy as they cause the mitochondria (energy centre of your cells) to swell and malfunction.
◆ They interfere with cell respiration and change the way your immune system works.
◆ They decrease testosterone, increase abnormal sperm, and interfere with pregnant animals.
◆ They correlate with low birth weight in human babies.
◆ They interfere with blood insulin function.
◆ They interfere with liver enzymes necessary for detoxification (the cytochrome P450 system).
◆ They change the fluidity of cell membranes, making them harder, slowing down their reactions, lowering cell vitality, and making cell membranes more leaky.
◆ They make platelets stickier.
◆ They increase the ratio of LDL (bad) cholesterol to HDL (good) cholesterol, increasing your chance of heart disease.
◆ Whenever you eat fat, it is incorporated directly into the walls of your cells. When trans-fatty acids are incorporated into the cell wall, the cell begins to lose control over what substances pass through the cell membrane into the cell, opening the doorway to salt, carcinogens, damaging free radicals, and chemicals from unnatural food sources. As they gradually accumulate within a cell, the cell becomes

susceptible to ultra-violet radiation and cancer. (Research shows that cooks who spend time wok or pan-frying have a higher incidence of lung cancer.)

♦ They also raise the level of Lp(a), the strongest known risk factor for cardiovascular disease. For more information visit www.rawperfection.co.uk

BEWARE – THEY ARE EVERYWHERE!

Trans-fatty acids (hydrogenated or partially hydrogenated oils) are widespread in our foods. You can find them in breads, cakes, cookies, crackers, digestive biscuits, breakfast cereals, instant soups, chocolate bars, desserts, fruit cakes, crisps, convenience and junk foods, peanuts and peanut butter. Even in the croutons used to make your healthy caesar salad. The law prohibits trans-fatty acids from being used in baby foods but not in yours, crazy isn't it!

Cooked fats clog up your blood, your arteries and lymphatic system and cause you to gain unnecessary excess weight. They are thick, heavy, have a deranged structure and are difficult for the body to process, metabolise and eliminate. Do you want them floating around your bloodstream?

UNLEASHING THE POWER OF LIPASE: DISSOLVING FATTY DEPOSITS

The most important lesson for you to learn about *raw* plant fats is that they can actually help strip your body of unwanted fat! The magical key that assists this natural process is the enzyme lipase – without it you'll gain unnecessary fat. The moment fat is cooked, lipase is destroyed, and fat devoid of lipase will accumulate in your body. When you introduce *raw* plant fats into your diet (avocados, nuts and seeds, olives) the cooked fat is metabolised, helping to prevent arteries or lymph fluid from blockage. When eaten, the fatty acids found in raw plant fats gradually begin to take the place of the cooked fatty acids occupying the cell membrane structure.

Research by Dr. Howell, author of Enzyme Nutrition and Udo Erasmus, author of Fats That Heal, Fats That Kill indicates that saturated and unsaturated fats are beneficial to health as long as they are raw. When enzymes are present, the structure of the fat is irrelevant!

ENZYME'S WORST ENEMY: THE PASSAGE OF TIME

Enzymes digest food, break down toxins, cleanse the blood, strengthen the immune system, build protein into muscle, assist in muscle contraction, eliminate carbon dioxide from the lungs, and reduce stress on the pancreas and other vital organs.

According to Dr Edward Howell, an 18 year-old body, produces 30 times more amylase (carbohydrate digesting enzymes) than a 69 year old. Dr Howell suggests if you eat an enzyme poor diet, you are inviting premature ageing. In fact the more lavishly a young body gives up its enzymes, the sooner the state of enzyme poverty or old age is reached. Are your eating habits increasing your enzyme supply or diminishing it?

♦ Enzyme function is suppressed in an acidic environment, so ensure you devour plenty of chlorophyll rich foods. Without active enzymes, intercellular activity begins to decline.

♦ Enzymes have as much of an impact on your health and well being as any other vital nutrient. Without them, vitamins, minerals, phytochemicals, proteins, fats and carbohydrates would be rendered useless! Enzymes activate vitamins and minerals. It's no use taking multiple supplements if you don't ensure your enzyme account is healthy.

♦ Enzymes are your body's labour force. Without them you'd be nothing more than a pile of lifeless chemicals.

♦ Enzyme rich foods help transform undigested food into its basic components. These are then absorbed and used to build cells, tissues and organs. They also form the basis of a healthy digestive system.

♦ When introduced directly into the bloodstream, enzymes tend to concentrate at the site of a wound, a tumour, inflammation, or immune system activity. Their ability to break down protein and fat molecules in various tissues of the body has been shown to reduce the size of blood clots and tumours, reduce inflammation, and speed tissue repair.

♦ Supplemental digestive enzymes can dramatically reduce inflammation and autoimmune activity in arthritis and other degenerative and inflammatory conditions.

♦ At body temperature, a tiny amount of pepsin (one of the gastric enzymes used to digest protein) will break down the white of an egg into small chain peptides within just a few minutes. To accomplish this feat in a laboratory would mean boiling the egg white for 24 hours in a

strong acid or alkali solution. That's the power of enzymes.
♦ As you increase the enzyme content of your diet, your bowel movements will become more regular, maybe more than twice a day.

CHOLECYSTOKININ: THE KEY TO SATISFACTION

As well as supplying an abundance of life-enhancing enzymes, raw plant fats cause the release of the hormone cholecystokinin (CKK) from the stomach that promotes satiety between meals. CCK goes directly to the brain to say, "Stop Eating." So in essence, raw plant fat is your primary hormonal off-switch for eating.

If you take the fat out of your diet and replace it with carbohydrate, you rob food of its taste and short circuit your "stop eating" hormone. In the process you'll crave more calories, over-stimulate the fat-storage-hormone insulin and find yourself on the slippery slope to obesity. Never underestimate the power of raw plant fats!

WHY FAT CAN HELP WITH FAT LOSS

In the 1950s, at the University of Middlesex in London, Professor Alan Kekwick and Dr. Gaston L.S. Pawan published a landmark study. They put patients on a diet that was low in calories (1000 calories) but 90% fat. What happened? The patients lost significant amounts of weight. When you read chapter 7 you'll learn that fat doesn't over-stimulate the fat-storage-hormone insulin, allowing you to eat more fat and actually lose weight, if that's your goal.

When the same patients were put on a diet where 90% of the calories came from carbohydrate and the calorie content remained consistent, there was virtually no weight loss. At the moment, virtually every so-called authority is discrediting dietary fat, and yet its advantages for a dieter never seem to be mentioned. Raw plant fat satiates the appetite. Raw plant fat stops carbohydrate craving. And fat, in the absence of carbohydrate, accelerates the burning of stored fat.

PREVENT THE CRAVING FOR COOKED FATS BY GRAZING

Galanin is the brain hormone that regulates your body's desire for fat. The more galanin you produce, the more fat you'll crave! Galanin is so powerful, that when injected into the hypothalamus of laboratory animals, they automatically select more fatty foods. To add insult to injury, the more galanin you produce, the more fat you store! If you ever get a craving for fat, don't use will power and force yourself to abstain, simply use raw plant fats to their advantage and eliminate the craving.

Another way to prevent unwanted fat cravings is to graze rather than gauge. Galanin is released when insulin levels drop very low. These times are usually between meals (when most people feel a desire to snack) or when people are crash dieting. If insulin levels do drop and the body begins to break down fat for energy, fat particles are released into the bloodstream and travel to the hypothalamus triggering the release of galanin. Eating more frequently and in smaller portions, causes the production of galanin to be cut and thus decreases fat cravings. Grazing also ensures your blood/insulin levels are as steady as a rock and this is the real key (raw plant fats also help to keep insulin levels stable by blunting insulin response. More about this later!) Fat was labelled the enemy at the end of the 20th Century, but the tables have turned, fat is now your friend, as long as it is raw!

RESTRICTION IS SYNONYMOUS WITH CRAVINGS

Most dieters fail because they eliminate chocolate, cakes, ice cream, sweets, butter, cheese etc. and their body begins to cry out for fat. Rather than eliminating anything from your diet, start to add all the foods that bring vitality and energy to your body (including raw plant fats) and gradually, your excellent habits will push out your old habits. Be patient. It'll happen, but at the same time...

AVOID LOW FAT, NO FAT COOKED PRODUCTS
THEY'RE A CRUEL JOKE!

Low fat, no fat products are a joke and usually taste no better than the packaging they are wrapped in! Not only are they cooked, but to give them taste, manufacturers load them with sugar, which your body turns into the same hard (saturated) fats, the avoidance of which was the reason for making the low fat, no fat foods in the first place. Crazy isn't it?

DELIVER POWERFUL BONE BUILDING MINERALS
TO YOUR BONES

You've already discovered the power of chlorophyll-rich greens, but if you want to maximise the absorption of the powerful bone building minerals found in green leafy vegetables, you must increase the use of raw plant fats. Studies show that raw plant fats act as a delivery vehicle for the minerals found in chlorophyll rich greens, helping your body to absorb calcium and deposit it in bone.

THE MAGIC OF THE AVOCADO

Avocados are marvellous! They should be at the heart of every diet. Not only will they prevent the cravings so often experienced when transitioning from a cooked diet to raw food diet, but they'll leave you full and satisfied. Treat them as your primary replacement for meat and dairy fat.

Avocados are a rich source of a monounsaturated fat called oleic acid. "We've found that these monounsaturated fats improve fat levels in the body and help control diabetes," says Abhimanyu Garg, M.D., associate professor of internal medicine and clinical nutrition at the University of Texas' South-western Medical Centre at Dallas.

The oleic acid in avocados can also create a favourable cholesterol level. In a study from Mexico, researchers compared the effects of two low-fat diets. The diets were the same except that one included avocados and the other didn't. Amazingly, by including this powerful food, LDL cholesterol was lowered, HDL cholesterol was raised and triglycerides were lowered. You couldn't get a more favourable cholesterol response. Avocados are also excellent at helping re-establish hormonal balance within the system:

♦ They also contain a seven-carbon sugar that depresses insulin production, making them an excellent choice for people with hypoglycaemia.
♦ One of the most important functions of raw plant fats is to slow the rate and speed of which sugars enter the digestive tract – blunting insulin response. If you've been sold on the idea of eating fruit only in the morning until noon, eat an avocado or two in the morning as

well. You'll benefit from a more sustained release of sugar into the bloodstream and thus more stable and more enduring energy levels.

Join the elite group of raw-foodists who eat between 2-5 avocados daily and enjoy clear smooth skin, stable energy levels and exceptional health. Avocados are also excellent sources of fibre, potassium and folate. Each of these nutrients are critical for optimal health. Take look why:

♦ One avocado contains 10 grams of fibre. That's more than a bran muffin and is 40% of your daily need.

♦ "You can never get too much potassium," says David B. Young, Ph.D., professor of physiology and biophysics at the University of Mississippi Medical Centre in Jackson. Avocados pack a huge potassium punch – about 1100mg, a third of your daily requirement. Studies indicate that people who eat diets high in potassium rich foods have a significantly lower risk of high blood pressure, heart attack and stroke.

♦ One avocado will also provide a third of your folate requirements, a nutrient that helps prevent life threatening birth defects of the brain and spine. All you potential mothers out there, take note! Folate is essential for keeping nerves functioning properly.

♦ Avocados, like all raw foods, are full of enzymes assisting your body in a multitude of ways.

♦ Use raw fat to your advantage when engineering hormonally perfect meals. Remember, the extra fat releases the hormone cholecystokinin (CKK), which promotes a feeling of fullness, slowing down the digestive process allowing you to feel fuller for longer.

THE ULTIMATE PROTEIN REPLACEMENT FOOD

It isn't protein your body needs to fill the space left by animal food, but raw plant fat. Even many nutritionists can't get this right! Fats are the all-important bridge between success and failure on an all-raw diet. Without fat you'll feel empty. Without fat you'll always want more. Without fat you'll never give your body what it instinctively desires. Choose your fat wisely. Choose raw plant fats and prepare to be satiated, full, and satisfied.

OLIVES: THE MOST POWERFUL MUCUS-DISSOLVING FRUIT IN ALL THE LAND

Olives are awesome. In a world where toxicity is rampant, you need as many foods as possible to remain toxin free. If a food has a high acid binding potential, it has a greater ability to dissolve mucus/cooked-food residues within the body. This is what makes olives so powerful for detoxification. They have the greatest propensity of any fruit to dissolve toxic mucus. The olive is the highest mucus dissolver of any fruit, having a rating of 30.56 on the mucus dissolving scale. Figs are close behind at 27.81. No other fruit ranks higher than 20. The orange, an excellent mucus dissolver, ranks at 9.61. See Ragnar Berg's food analysis table in the appendix for a further explanation.

The olive is also the bodybuilding food of the gods. Stephen Arlin is a body builder and author of Raw Power. He eats raw food exclusively and at 6ft 2inches tall, maintains a muscle filled body weighing in at 226lbs. He calls olives his 'dianabol' (dianabol is an illegal steroid, often used by bodybuilders to make rapid 'gains' in size and strength). If you want a food that is going to saturate your body with muscle building, life-enhancing elements, olives are a must for you. Take a look why:

- Olives have the highest mineral content of any fruit.
- Olives contain twice as much calcium as oranges by weight, making them the most potent fruit source of calcium.
- Olives are high in magnesium.
- Olives are an excellent source of amino acids, including: leucine, aspartic acid, and glutamic acid.
- Olives are a fatty fruit helping stimulate CCK and eliminating cravings.
- Olives are loaded with beneficial omega 3 and omega 6 fatty acids, needed for eicosanoid production.
- Olives are high in vitamins A and E.
- Olives are antioxidant powerhouses, which help to deactivate free radicals.
- Olives are able to soothe the mucous membranes with its oil.

STONE PRESSED OLIVE OIL – A NUTRITIONAL GOLD-MINE

Some olive oils are devoid of lipase (the fat-splitting enzyme), because they are made from unripe olives. I recommend only organic stone-crushed, cold pressed extra virgin olive oil in dark bottles (oils are light sensitive). Olive oil is a soothing fat for damaged and dry skin, hair, and nails. It can be used to soothe the skin after shaving. Olive oil may be used on baby skin instead of the harsh 'baby oil' brands available in stores.

THE PHYTOCHEMICAL REVOLUTION: MINOR INGREDIENTS FROM MAGICAL OILS

Whether you choose to eat more sprouted nuts and seeds or consume stone pressed oils or both, your health will benefit from the minor ingredients (phytochemicals) that make up about 2% of the oils. Phytochemicals are nature's pharmacy and must remain in foods if they are to create optimal health.

Minor ingredients found in various unrefined seed and nut oils can:
♦ Lower cholesterol, and block cholesterol absorption from foods.
♦ Improve cardiovascular function.
♦ Improve digestion, and stimulate pancreatic enzyme production.
♦ Improve liver and gall bladder function, and increase bile flow.
♦ Act as anti-oxidants and stabilise essential fatty acids against oxidation (rancidity).
♦ Act as anti-inflammatory agents.
♦ Protect visual functions, and improve brain (CNS) function.

Hundreds of different phytochemicals are found in different oils. The health benefits of traditional extra virgin (green) olive oil are based on phytochemicals.

DON'T GO TOO NUTS ABOUT NUTS – NIBBLE THEM!

If you eat a lot of nuts or feel it is a good way to increase more raw fat into your diet, make sure you abide by the following rules:

- Nuts are acid forming. If you experience a mucus discharge from your nose, it is just your body's way of dispelling acid forming minerals, in an effort to create a more alkaline environment.
- Eat nuts moderately (a maximum of 0.33 pounds or 0.15 kg per day). Put your daily ration in a tub every morning, this will prevent you from overeating them.
- Never eat more than 2.0-2.5 pounds (0.9-1.2kg) of nuts per week
- Balance nuts with green leafed vegetables and juicy sweet fruits.
- Take a break from nuts every month or so for a few days or a week.
- Soak nuts and seeds for a minimum of 8 hours to disarm their enzyme inhibitors.
- If eaten in the dormant state without green leaves to help digestion, nuts and seeds can burden the pancreas and sit "heavy" in the stomach.
- Choose brazil, almonds, hazelnuts, macadamia, pecans, pistachio, walnuts and pine nuts.
- Macadamia nuts have the most fat and the least protein of all nuts.
- Cashews are usually cooked in order to release them from their shell. Steer clear of cashews unless you can guarantee they're raw.
- Use nuts to provide a dense fat substance that moves into the lymph and thickens your tissues – this protects you from city pollution. If you are totally purified on a raw-food diet containing little or no fat, pollution can filter into you (particles move from areas of greater concentration to areas of lesser concentration).
- Nut fats are a rich source of antioxidants, helping to protect you against free radicals/city toxins.

LIGHTEN THE LOAD ON YOUR LIVER

If you have any form of liver damage, choose lighter fats such as avocados or blended seeds instead of heavy fats such as nuts. You'll learn to realise when you've eaten more fat than your liver can handle, so pay attention! Usually, when your liver is working hard processing raw plant fats, your appetite will shut down.

THE CHOICE IS ALL YOURS:
SELECTING THE FINEST RAW PLANT FATS

Here is a selection of the best raw plant fats. Add these to your shopping list:

Akee (a relative of the durian fruit found growing in West Africa and the West Indies), avocados, borage seed oil, coconut butter (consume 3-4 tablespoons each day if possible), durians, grape seeds, hemp seed and its oil, nuts of all types (except cashews), raw nut butters (almond butter is excellent), olives and their oil (stone pressed if possible), pumpkin seeds and their oil (cold pressed), sesame seeds, sunflower seeds, Tahini (sesame butter), unhulled Tahini (an alkaline fat, high in calcium), young coconuts (available at Asian markets).

ARE YOU READY FOR THE CHALLENGE?

Raw plant fats are critical! You must include them in your diet and avoid all cooked fats. Use raw plant fats to bridge the gap from a cooked food lifestyle to a raw food existence. Although fats have been seen as the enemy for many years, raw plant fats are your closest friends. Respect them, use them to your advantage and reap the rewards...

- Raw plant fats absorb sunlight, increasing their oxygen reacting ability a 1000 times, making them very chemically active.
- Raw plant fats help carry toxins and other substances to the surface of your skin, intestinal tract, kidneys, or lungs where these substances are discarded. The slight negative charge carried by raw plant fats allows them to do this. They disperse concentrations of substances, causing them to spread out in a very thin layer over surfaces. This charge also prevents each molecule from aggregating as they repel one another.
- Raw plant fats hold oxygen in the cell membranes where they prevent foreign organisms such as viruses and bacteria entering by creating a barrier. Such organisms cannot thrive in the presence of oxygen.
- Raw plant fats are the precursors of a gang of hormone-like substances known as eicosanoids. These short-lived substances regulate virtually every function in your body. See chapter 8.
- Raw plant fats are the precursors of the highly active, very highly unsaturated fatty acids required for brain cells, synapses, retina, adrenal

glands, and testes to function properly.

♦ Raw plant fats improve performance by improving calmness under pressure and improving your ability to concentrate. They also help you sleep better and decrease your sleep requirement. Lack of raw plant fats causes weakness and clumsiness.

♦ Raw plant fats improve performance because they improve the capacity of your liver and kidneys for detoxification. They also enhance the ability of glands such as the thyroid. Every gland needs its supply of raw plant fats.

♦ Raw plant fats improve performance by improving gut integrity, allowing you to digest and absorb nutrients more efficiently. They help prevent energy-robbing allergic reactions secondary to poor digestion. They also help you maintain a healthy intestinal flora promoting the growth of friendly microorganisms in your intestines and prevent the unfriendly ones from thriving.

♦ In your immune system, raw plant fats protect your genetic material (DNA) from damage. Omega 3 essential fatty acids have anti-oxidant-like functions in the oil soluble system of your body (similar to the anti-oxidant functions of vitamin C in the water-soluble system). Their anti-oxidant ability also protects you from the damaging effects of free radicals. Your immune cells use raw plant fats to make oxygen 'bullets' to kill infectious foreign invaders preventing them from eating your tissues.

♦ Raw plant fats protect you from the toxic influences of oil-soluble pollutants such as pesticides, PCBs and chlorinated hydrocarbons. These oil-soluble poisons exit your body with the oil.

♦ Raw plant fats help treat fungus infections like athlete's foot and yeast over growth (candida). They've also been known to inhibit tumour growth.

♦ Raw plant fats elevate mood and lift depression – a reason why some people overeat. Elevated mood and increased energy levels also make us feel like being active.

♦ Raw plant fats help prevent cravings of all kinds.

♦ Raw plant fats help your kidneys dump excess water, decreasing unnecessary bloating. Without them, your kidneys cannot do their job properly and you'll retain water in your tissues.

♦ Raw plant fats lower the glycemic index of sweet and starchy foods, dampening the insulin response of high glycemic foods.

♦ Raw plant fats make skin soft, smooth and velvety, and are excellent internal, edible cosmetics. The best way to oil the skin is from within. You'll tan better, burn less, get relief from eczema, acne, psoriasis, and other skin conditions.

♦ Sperm formation requires essential fatty acids. In the female reproductive cycle, they help prevent pre-menstrual syndrome.

♦ Raw plant fats contain an abundance of antioxidants that deactivate free radicals by giving them electrons. The spare electrons in fats help sweep toxins along to the liver. In a healthy body, when there are spare electrons, ageing is slowed.

♦ Donald Rudin, MD, showed that when juvenile delinquents were given omega 3 rich oils, they became more responsive to counselling. The human brain is made from food, and requires essential fatty acids to function, it's up to us as parents to take responsibility and feed our children raw plant fats. Lead by example.

FEROCIOUS ENERGY, PERFORMANCE AND STAYING POWER WITH RAW PLANT FATS

When athletes balance their essential fatty acid intake, their performance both in strength and in endurance increases dramatically. Whether you are a world-class athlete, amateur enthusiast or visit a health-club regularly, you need to include the right kind of fat in your diet to increase recovery time and enhance performance. Take a closer look:

♦ Raw plant fats improve performance by making red blood cell membranes more flexible, allowing them to slide through your capillaries more easily, which in turn improves the delivery of nutrients and oxygen to your cells, tissues, organs, glands and muscles.

♦ Raw plant fats attract oxygen like a magnet! Raw plant fats are involved with the transfer of oxygen from the air in the lungs – through the alveolar membrane – through the capillary wall – into the blood plasma – across the membranes of the red blood cells – to the haemoglobin – to all cells in the body. They make oxygen available to the tissues, by activating oxygen molecules.

♦ Raw plant fats help you recover from fatigue quicker, because recovery requires oxygen, and essential fatty acids increase the body's ability to metabolise oxygen.

♦ Raw plant fats help you to lose unwanted body fat by increasing the rate at which you burn calories. They make you feel more energetic and therefore more physically active. Refusal to exercise is usually due to lack of energy. Raw plant fats provide that energy, where as cooked fats make you feel lazy and lethargic and slow your metabolic rate.

♦ Raw plant fats keep you slim. They are also anabolic and decrease recovery time of fatigued muscles after exercise, by facilitating the conversion of lactic acid to water and carbon dioxide. If you workout with weights you'll perform better, grow faster and recover quicker. (Combine raw plant fats with green leafy vegetables after a workout for excellent results.)

♦ Raw plant fats are anti-catabolic. They are part of protein metabolism, and prevent muscle breakdown. Without raw plant fats, protein can become toxic (a warning for those who eat lots of protein to build muscles and avoid fats because they have been misinformed by those with a rampant fat phobia).

♦ Raw plant fats are required for testosterone production and insulin function, both of which are important for muscular development. Body builders on low fat diets fail to gain the development they strive for, because testosterone is required for muscle development.

♦ Raw plant fats have anti-inflammatory properties. They help minimise joint, tendon and ligament strain.

In 1900, deaths from cardiovascular disease accounted for only 15% of all deaths from all causes. But today, 100 years later, with an increase of over 350%, it kills over 50% of the entire population. In 1900, cancer killed 1 person in every 30. Today it kills over 1 in 4 of the entire population. So much for medical advances! If you were to chart the increases in disease from other forms of fatty degeneration such as diabetes, multiple sclerosis, kidney degeneration and liver degeneration you'd find similar increases. Tissue and blood levels of people with diseases of fatty degeneration (Cardiovascular disease, cancer, diabetes, arthritis, obesity, mental dysfunction) are low in essential fatty acids. When essential fatty acids are added to the diets of these people, the symptoms surrounding the diseases begin to fade. When fat is cooked, diseases and deaths prevail. Be warned!

THE RAW PERFECTION EVALUATION
Do you happily eat a variety of raw plant fats?
Have you eliminated cooked fat from your diet?

The world can be a harsh place. Toxicity is everywhere and nutritionally void foodstuffs seem to be becoming more and more common place. The result: Your body becomes a filter as toxicity begins to drain you of your energy and vitality. There is a simple answer...

CHAPTER 5

DETOXIFICATION: SPARKLING FROM THE INSIDE OUT

Health is as infectious as disease, given the right conditions for its spread –
Dr George Scott-Williamson, 1943

The current perception of detoxification is a nightmare! People tend to think they have to be on a detoxification diet for detoxification to occur. Wrong! Detoxification is a process that is occurring in your body every minute of every day as your body removes unnecessary obstructions in an attempt to restore health and vitality. Whenever waste matter passes out of your body via your skin, bowels, urine, breath etc. you are ridding your body of waste. This is the natural process of detoxification and by embracing it, you'll begin to eliminate waste faster and embrace exuberant health. If you suppress detoxification, the build up of obstructions can rob you of your health and invite early death. Harsh, but true! Every natural process in your body is designed to preserve life. If you don't assist the detoxification process you'll never eliminate the obstructions that can eventually lead to your demise.

BEGIN RESTRUCTURING YOUR BODY TODAY!

Today you have the opportunity to make a very important decision. Over the course of the next two years, 98% of the atoms in your body will be completely replaced! Over the course of the next seven years, 100% of your body will be replaced! You are constantly recreating yourself out of the food, air and water you ingest.

If you make the decision to fully detoxify, you'll have to battle with detoxification, struggle with symptoms of past illnesses, and learn to handle criticism from your peers. If you embrace the journey, it'll be one of the most rewarding ever taken. Ultimately you'll have the joy of knowing that every cell and atom in your body is crackling with energy and built from something alive and vibrant. Whether you're in your teens or about to reach 100, it's never too late to regenerate.

THE TUBES OF DETOXIFICATION

The best way to think of detoxification, intoxication and digestion is to imagine that your body consists of three layers of 'tubes'.

1. The first tube is your digestive system. It runs from your mouth to your anus and consists of the mouth, oesophagus, stomach, intestines, and colon. Each of these organs help to break down and assimilate foods.
2. The second tube is your circulatory system and it draws in whatever is present in the first tube. If you've just ingested E3Live for example, the chlorophyll, enzymes, amino acids, vitamins, minerals, phytochemicals and trace elements will enter your bloodstream ready to create amazing health. If you've eaten a meal of cooked meat and pasteurised milk, your bloodstream will draw in those elements and your blood will thicken and slow down. The second tube consists of arteries, veins, capillaries, and the heart.
3. The third tube is the lymphatic system. It bathes all the organs, muscles, bodily tissues and cells, and draws in whatever is present in the bloodstream in order to feed every cell in your body. If the bloodstream is full of powerful nutrients, the cells will get a good feed. If the bloodstream is full of the waste associated with a meal containing milk and meat, the cells will be poorly nourished.

The lymphatic system also returns the waste products of cell metabolism back to the blood and back to the intestines. The goal of detoxification is to keep the bloodstream clean and full of vital nutrients, so the lymph fluid can mobilise the waste that it has built up around the cells before eliminating it.

Did you know that you have four times as much lymph in your body as you do blood? It's the lymph fluid that bathes every cell, drawing nutrients (and waste) from the bloodstream before delivering them to the cells.

Detoxification is easy to understand if you remember the concept of diffusion from chemistry class. The principle of diffusion states that molecules move from an area of greater concentration to an area of lesser concentration. Detoxification begins when the blood is thinner than the lymph fluid, allowing trapped toxicity in the lymph to diffuse back into the blood to be eliminated. When you begin to eat more raw foods, your blood will thin out and any toxic undigested molecules trapped in your lymph fluid will begin to enter your bloodstream. The importance of thinning the blood naturally cannot be overstated. The cleaner you keep your blood, the quicker the lymphatic system will be able to release stored toxins. Eventually, there will be no more toxins left in the lymphatic system leaving only room for remarkable health.

To illustrate this, watch the video by Dr. Michael Klaper, entitled 'A Diet For All Reasons'. Dr. Klaper shows you the effects of a typical cooked meat and pasteurised milk diet on the bloodstream. After only a few hours of ingesting this waste, the blood becomes very thick and heavy! Is that the picture of health you want for yourself? Is that what you want flowing around your veins and arteries?

Did you know that there are more heart attacks in the United States on Thanksgiving Day than any other day of the year?

SURGEONS KNOW THIS – WHY DON'T YOU?

Did you know that surgeons refuse to operate on a patient unless they've fasted on water for at least 8 hours? They know from first hand experience the dangers involved when the bloodstream isn't flowing freely enough. Cooked foods insulate and dampen your body's electrical nervous system. Senses become dulled and life becomes grey rather than colourful. The message: Choose to eat raw foods and thin your blood naturally.

LET YOUR BLOOD FLOW FREELY
WITH GARLIC AND ONIONS

If you suspect heavy detoxification symptoms, include garlic and onions in your diet. They both thin the blood naturally. Obstructions such as cooked fat, cooked protein and other toxins pass easily into the lymph during detoxification, making the blood very thick, sometimes even causing blood pressure to rise, due to an obstructed circulatory system.

Be warned – You may feel worse before you feel better! If your diet has been full of cooked foods, I suggest you take it easy. Begin by slowly increasing the amount of raw food in your diet whilst exercising regularly. If your diet was generally healthy and was abundant in many raw foods anyway, go for it!

It takes years for your tissues to become clogged by toxicity, and in the same way, takes years to dissolve, dislodge and eliminate these materials. On a raw diet you can expect it to take as many months to detoxify your body as it has years you've been alive. If you're 50 years old, it may take 50 months to completely eliminate all the waste.

LYMPHOLOGISTS DISCOVER
A DEADLY CAUSE OF DEATH!

After months of investigation and research, Dr. C Samuel West, chemist and lymphologist, concluded that: "If blood proteins cannot be removed from the spaces around the cells by the lymphatic system, they can cause death within just a few hours."

Can you see the importance of eating foods that don't obstruct your bloodstream? By consciously doing all you can to keep your bloodstream thin, these obstructions will eventually be eliminated from your lymph fluid, opening the doorway for exceptional health.

If you want your lymph to be clean and toxin free, your bloodstream needs to be clean and toxin free. If you want your bloodstream to be clean and toxin free you need to eat a diet that is clean and toxin free. Fruits, raw plant fats and green leafy vegetables should take pride of place in your diet. You'll find that over a period of time, your body will change in front of your eyes, from a solid, rigid, weakened condition, to a free, elastic, fluid, and energetic condition. The importance of stretching, Yoga, Pilates, aerobic exercise, and massage cannot be overstated as each of these speed up the process of elimination by stimulating the circulation of blood and lymphatic fluid.

BURNING PARASITES OUT OF YOUR BODY WITH RIPE HOP PEPPERS

Commercial meat is loaded with parasitic worms, giving you a good reason to eliminate all animal products from your diet immediately. Parasites feed on toxicity, especially cooked starch and animal protein. If you want to eliminate parasites or take a preventative measure in keeping them at bay, take your pick from garlic, onion, ripe hot peppers, ginger, radishes, etc. and ensure you eat them regularly. Ripe hot foods are invaluable to health. Not only do they burn parasites out of your intestines but they also stimulate the intestines. It's important to know that parasites can prevent weight gain and cause emaciation.

Natural Hygienists are against ripe hot foods, claiming they irritate the body! They are right, but the fact is they irritate the parasites within the body! Hot peppers are excellent foods to eat if you live in the city. Every city has its fair share of people who are either ill or very toxic. If you live in the city, you are likely to come into contact with these people on a moment-to-moment basis. Hot peppers are antibiotic, wiping out harmful bacteria and boosting your immune system. The hot nature of these foods may prompt you to eat them with foods that dampen the heat such as avocados or nuts. If hot peppers are too strong, try garlic, onions or ginger as an alternative.

PROTECT YOURSELF AGAINST POLLUTION WITH RAW PLANT FATS

Symptoms of detoxification disappear the moment you eat something cooked because as soon as the blood is thickened, toxins begin re-entering the lymph fluid rather than exiting. Remember the law of diffusion? The best way to remain on an all-raw diet whilst slowing the detoxification process is to eat raw plant fats such as young coconuts, avocados, nuts and seeds with green-leafed vegetables. This is also a great strategy to prevent environmental pollution from entering your body. If you live in the city and thicken your blood with raw plant fats, you won't act as a filter for 'city pollution'. If your bloodstream is free of toxicity and thin, pollution (toxicity) will move from areas of greater concentration (the city) into areas of lower concentration (your blood and body)! Be warned!

ELECTRIFY YOUR BLOOD AND SUPERCHARGE YOUR BODY WITH CHLOROPHYLL RICH GREENS

Raw greens are powerful! They alkalise your blood and increase your blood's electricity. With increased electricity, your blood becomes more soluble allowing it to suspend, metabolise or eliminate more undigested and misappropriated minerals. As you already know through your knowledge of wheatgrass juice and E3Live, chlorophyll and the alkaline compounds found in green leafy vegetables/AFA algae can combine with heavy metals, allowing for their rapid elimination. If you know of anyone with heavy metal poisoning, persuade them to use E3Live and natural green juices immediately.

FRUIT: THE KINGS OF CLEANSING

If you've ever been concerned about the water purity in your immediate environment, worry no more! Fruit is one of the finest sources of biologically purified water you'll ever find. Sweet fruits have also captured nutrients from the sun and are relentless cleansers and mucus dissolvers. One of the most effective ways of cleansing your body of toxicity is to eat a diet high in water-content fruit. Their high carbon content encourages them to act as incinerators of waste matter in the digestive system, bloodstream, internal organs and skin. Fruit also has a high potassium content, which is helpful in ridding your system and tissues of excess water, increasing oxygenation in the cells.

PINEAPPLE'S POWERFUL DETOXIFYING ENZMES SPEED UP PROTEIN DIGESTION

Pineapple is a concentrated source of bromelain, an enzyme that activates the hydrochloric acid in your stomach and helps to break down any undigested protein. Pineapple is also believed to soothe internal inflammation, accelerate tissue repair, stimulate hormone production and clear away mucus in the gut. If your diet has been full of concentrated sources of protein such as eggs, fish, meat and foul, eat pineapple to help eliminate these foods. Pawpaw and mango are rather expensive but rich in the enzyme papain. Papain resembles the enzyme pepsin in the stomach and like bromelain, helps to break down excess protein. Both fruits are good for cleansing the intestines.

FOLLOW IN THE FOOTSTEPS OF YOUR EARLY ANCESTORS

Dr Alan Walker, an eminent anthropologist at John Hopkins University, found that early ancestors lived primarily on a diet of fruit. They were not predominantly meat eaters or even gatherers of seeds, shoots, leaves and grasses. They weren't omnivorous either. This conclusion was made by studying the striations on the fossilised teeth of early specimens and by examining the contents of fossilised intestines. Take a look for yourself at the amazing power of fruit and you'll see why it must make up a healthy portion of your diet:

♦ Fruit is 80 to 90% water content and residing within the water is every vital element necessary for maximum cleansing and elimination, including minerals, vitamins, enzymes, phytochemicals, fibres, carbohydrates, amino acids and fatty acids.

♦ Fruit requires less energy to digest than any other food, demanding practically none! Most foods spend anywhere between 1.5 – 4 hours in the stomach, but fruits are pre-digested and pass through an empty stomach in only 20 – 30 minutes. Ensure you always eat fruit on an empty stomach or it will sit on top of the previous meal and ferment, causing bloating and wind!

♦ The high carbon content of fruit causes them to be powerful detoxifiers and incinerators of waste material.

♦ Fruit also has a high potassium content, ridding your body of excess water and strengthening the micro-electrical potentials within cells.

♦ The value of a high fruit diet cannot be overstated, especially in sickness, ill health, or whenever the body is filled with poisons. Germs cannot grow and live in fruit juices. Typhoid fever and cholera germs cannot resist the action of fruit juices such as lemon, orange, pineapple, strawberry, apple, and grapefruit. A high fruit diet will disinfect the stomach and alimentary canal.

♦ When the sugar in fruit enters your bloodstream it affects the saturation centre in the hypothalamus of your brain, satisfying your appetite almost immediately.

♦ The Harvard School of Public Health demonstrated that a higher fibre intake correlates with an increased chance of maintaining stable insulin levels. Elements present in soluble fibre such as guars and pectins form a gummy gel that lines the intestine and slows absorption of glucose. Choose apples to begin your day since they have a lot of pectin.

♦ The amount of fruit you eat per meal should not exceed 500 – 600 grams, but better still is to graze through the day eating one piece fruit, every 1 – 2 hours. Make sure you wait at least 30mins before eating any other foods after eating a piece of fruit. If you've eaten a banana, wait an hour.

♦ With its sweet blends of rare flavours, delightful aromas, and eye pleasing colours, eating fruit is always a pleasurable experience.

♦ Eat as many different kinds of fruit as you can over a weeklong period. There's no boiling, no steaming, no frying, no baking – just 'eat and go!' Use them for what they are, one of the most important foods in your RAW PERFECTION arsenal.

Start your day with fruit. Your stomach is empty, so break your overnight fast (break-fast) with the only food that is going to set you up for a day of vibrancy. Use avocados and olives to add valuable raw fat to your diet and help slow the rate of carbohydrate entry into your blood. This way you'll enjoy stable energy levels. You can make life as easy as possible for yourself, or you can struggle through it. Fruit makes life effortless, giving you the abundance you need.

FROM YOUR BLOODSTREAM TO YOUR CELLS:
THE NEVER ENDING INTERCHANGE OF CHEMICALS AND ENERGY

Most cells are protected from the bloodstream by a group of cells called endothelial cells. These cells determine what substances enter and exit the cell. If you have a toxic body, nutrients and hormones are sometimes prevented from entering a target cell, because the endothelial cells are obstructed with toxic waste matter. If you read a lot of best-selling nutritional books these days, you'll find a lot of talk about hormones. The importance of eating a diet that promotes a healthy balance of various hormones for optimal health is critical, but if your body is full of toxicity...

COMMUNICATION BETWEEN
YOUR HORMONES AND CELLS SUFFERS

Scientists from the University of Vienna were able to show that raw food nutrition is the only method that can systematically help in eliminating the sticky marsh that surrounds cells (the result of a diet that includes sticky cooked starches and cooked meat).

As the sticky marsh is gradually eliminated the ability of capillaries to regulate the transportation of nutrients and hormones is optimised. Once the waste is cleared from the cells, the sodium/potassium balance inside and outside the cells is restored.

SUGAR PUTS THE BREAKS ON DETOXIFICATION

Another reason to eliminate cooked convenience food from your diet is sugar! Sugar found in many cooked/convenience foods inhibits the production of the enzymes needed for the detoxification process, weakening liver function. Once you've eliminated sugar, you'll want to strengthen your production of the detoxifying liver enzymes and to do so include lots of cruciferous vegetables in your diet. An excellent source is kale as it is high in a substance called sulforaphane. Sulforaphane helps your liver convert toxins into non-toxic wastes that can then be removed from your body.

PREPARING FOR SHORT-TERM PAIN
TO ACHIEVE LONG-TERM GAIN

As you unburden your lymph of undigested proteins, toxins and unwanted chemicals, you may experience any number of short-term symptoms of detoxification. Take a look at these symptoms and prepare yourself – It could be you!

Fevers, diarrhoea, desires for poor foods, tastes of old medicines, mucus discharges, bad breath, coughs, cold symptoms, drowsiness, momentary aches, nausea, unclear thinking, weight loss, intestinal discomfort, gas, headaches, light-headedness, rashes, cloudy urine, swelling of the feet, dryness and itching of the skin and scalp.

To eliminate all this unwanted waste from your body, your body will make use of all the eliminative organs, including your bowels, mouth, sinuses, skin, and kidneys. A great indicator is your urine. If it is clear, your blood is clean (at that moment). If it is dark or cloudy then your body is releasing toxins.

You may also experience emotional detoxification, where emotions such as anxiety, depression, and other imbalances expel themselves from your body. If you experience any of these symptoms, feel delighted that you've had the courage to see the process through to the end. I send you my congratulations.

CREATING A PASSAGE TO BE PROUD OF!

Once you've begun the journey into the kingdom of raw foods, book an appointment with a colon hydrotherapist. Colonic hydrotherapy is a gentle internal bath using warm, purified water that can help to eliminate stored faecal matter, gas, mucus and toxic substances from the colon. Once the colon is clean and more efficient, detoxification and elimination will be enhanced, laying the foundation for exceptional health.

Did you know that the transit time of food through your body should be less than 24 hours? On average in the UK it is now 60 hours for men and 70 for women. The United Kingdom is the most constipated nation in the world and has the highest incidence of bowel cancer in the world with 20,000 new cases every year.

Unless you are sick, I don't believe it is a good idea to completely clean your colon with a series of colonics until you've established excellent eating habits. Once your diet is predominantly green leafy vegetables and their juices, raw plant fats, fruits and sprouts then colonic irrigation is a must!

**"I WOULD TRAVEL 1000 MILES FOR SOME COLONICS BEFORE I WOULD ALLOW MYSELF TO BE TAKEN TO HOSPITAL"
– DR NORMAN WALKER, AUTHOR OF COLON HEALTH**

If you've never had a colonic or a series of them, don't be led to believe that only one will be enough. You should take as many as you can until the colon is perfectly clean. Once your colon is thoroughly cleaned, you will experience a magical state of health. Combine this with excellent eating habits and you'll want to have a series of irrigations twice a year, to maintain optimal health.

If you suffer from any of the following afflictions, you must book a series of colonics today. It'll be the best money you've ever spent.

Constipation, fatigue, poor eyesight, hearing loss, asthma, prostate trouble, colds, allergies, nagging back ache, respiratory disorders, excessive gas, abdominal pain, colitis, thyroid deficiency, diabetes, hayfever, tonsilitus, sore throat, chest problems, glandular problems, heart problems, liver difficulties, gall bladder problems, over-exhausted pancreas and breast lumps.

There is no ailment, sickness or disease that cannot or will not respond to treatment quicker and more effectively. My recommendation is that twice a year, throughout the rest of your life you have a colonic or a series of colonics to maintain a perfectly clean colon. Your health depends on it. Your life depends on it!

WHEN YOUR COLON IS COMPLETELY CLEAN YOUR HEALTH WILL BE REVITALISED

Imagine working as a colon hydrotherapist and seeing 100 patients with hay fever walk through your door. Imagine giving them all a series of colonics and finding that every last patient was 'cured' from their symptoms! You may think it strange to blame the symptoms of hay fever, a runny nose and sore throat on the condition of the colon, but nearly everyone who has experienced colonic irrigation has benefited from complete remission. Dr Norman walker states in his book Colon Health that every X-ray taken of a hay fever sufferer shows trouble in exactly the same area of the colon.

Even those who have been advised to go under the knife of the surgeon for breast removal (due to lumps being found in the breast tissue) have found that after a series of colonic irrigations, the lumps completely disappeared in a matter of days!

THE GOLDEN RULE:
DETOXIFICATION, LIKE INTOXICATION,
IS A STEP BY STEP PROCESS

If you experience various discomforts when you transition from a cooked diet to a raw diet, and 'appear' to be wasting away, be patient. Know within yourself that as long as you are eating an abundance of green leafy vegetables, raw plant fats and fruit/juices your body will soon begin glowing from the inside out. Nature takes its own time, it doesn't repair years of bad habits overnight – Be patient! Eventually you will gain weight until your perfect body weight is attained. You may even become heavier! Obesity occurs when the unnatural part of you (or 'false body' – as some people call it) is growing out of control.

REJUVENATE YOUR BODY
WITH SAUNA DETOXIFICATION

A gentleman in America spent the best part of his working life surrounded by diesel fuel and exhaust fumes. He experienced constant migraine headaches, varying sickness, had achy joints and was so allergic to most modern buildings and appliances that he was considering moving to the desert! Fortunately a close friend told him about a sauna detoxification centre and the gentleman checked in.

When the gentleman began the program, the detoxification process was so powerful, the others in the sauna were forced to leave because the fumes leaving his body were so toxic! Eventually the centre built a special exhaust vent to expel the fumes out of the building! That's how powerful the detoxification process can be!

SPARKLING FROM THE INSIDE OUT

Once you've eliminated the toxins from your body, the future automatically becomes bright and inspiring. Here's what you've got to look forward to:

♦ Increased endurance and energy, faster reflexes and increased sexual vigour.
♦ Only 4-6 hours of sleep required each night.

- Greater concentration, improved memory and mental focus, clearer more logical thinking and increased creativity.
- Fresher breath, decreased body odour, a better sense of smell and hearing, and improved eyesight.
- Elimination of pollen and animal allergies and the ability to breathe deeper and hold your breath longer.
- Increased resistance to hot and cold weather and invulnerability to sunburn.
- Quick and strong growth of hair and fingernails.
- Controlled temper, decreased stress, and increased confidence.
- The ability to fast with no adverse side effects.
- Increased individualism, a superior attitude towards life, nature, and the order of things, and a closer relationship with natural forces.

ARE YOU READY FOR THE CHALLENGE?

Increasing the amount of raw food you eat in your diet is an excellent starting point. Balancing raw plant fats, green leafy vegetables and fruits is another critical step, but the biggest challenge you'll ever face is that of complete detoxification. Start small and get used to eating raw meals and simple foods. If you have an undiminished belief that raw nutrition is the only normal and natural way to live, I congratulate you. I had to read many books, talk to others and use my body as the experimental laboratory. My belief in nature is now strong enough to carry me through the cyclical lows of the detoxification process. Here's a re-cap:

- Detoxification is something that is going on in your body all the time. If you embrace this natural process and assist it, you'll eliminate waste faster, remove obstructions from your body and allow exuberant health to emerge
- Over the next two years, 98% of the atoms in your body will be completely replaced! Over the next seven years, 100% of your body will be replaced! Detoxify and eliminate the waste, setting the foundation for the ultimate re-build.
- You have in your body approximately 1.2 gallons (4.5 litres) of blood, but four times as much lymph fluid.
- Lymph bathes every cell, drawing nutrients (and waste) from the bloodstream, and delivering them to the cells.
- Imagine that your body consists of three layers of 'tubes', your

digestive system, your circulatory system and your lymphatic system. Detoxification begins as soon as the blood is thinner than the lymph fluid, allowing trapped toxicity in the lymph to diffuse back into the blood to be eliminated.

♦ The cleaner you keep your blood, the quicker the lymphatic system will be able to release stored toxins, leaving room for exceptional health.

♦ A typical cooked meat and pasteurised milk diet leaves the blood thick and heavy.

♦ There are more heart attacks in the United States on Thanksgiving Day than any other day of the year.

♦ Surgeons won't operate on a patient unless they've fasted on water for at least 8 hours because of the dangers involved when the bloodstream isn't flowing freely enough.

♦ Garlic and onions thin the blood naturally.

♦ You may feel worse before you feel better when detoxifying, especially if your old diet was full of non-nutritional cooked food.

♦ It takes years for your tissues to become clogged by toxicity and in the same way takes years to dissolve, dislodge and eliminate these materials.

♦ On a raw diet you can expect it to take as many months to detoxify your body as it has years you've been alive. If you're 50 years old, it may take 50 months to completely eliminate all the waste.

♦ The importance of stretching, Yoga, Pilates, exercise, and massage cannot be overstated as each of these speed up the process of elimination by stimulating the circulation of blood and lymphatic fluid.

♦ Raw greens alkalise your blood and increase your blood's electricity, allowing it to become more soluble and thus suspend, metabolise or eliminate more undigested and misappropriated minerals.

♦ Choose wheatgrass juice and E3Live. The chlorophyll and the alkaline compounds in green leafy vegetables/AFA algae can combine with heavy metals, allowing for their rapid elimination.

♦ Ripe hot foods burn parasites out of your intestines. Parasites can prevent weight gain and cause emaciation. Use garlic, onion, ripe hot peppers, ginger etc.

♦ If you live in the city and thicken your blood with raw plant fats, you won't act as a filter for 'city pollution'. If your bloodstream is incredibly clean, pollution (toxicity) will move from areas of greater concentration (the city) into areas of lower concentration (your body)! Be warned!

- Sweet Fruits have captured nutrients from the sun and are relentless cleansers and mucus dissolvers. The high carbon content encourages them to act as incinerators of waste matter in the digestive system, the bloodstream, the internal organs and the skin.
- Scientists from the University of Vienna proved that raw food nutrition is the best method for eliminating the sticky marsh that surrounds cells, optimising nutrient and hormone transportation and restoring optimal sodium/potassium balance inside and outside of cells.
- The healthy transit time of food through your body should be less than 24 hours. On average in the UK it is now between 60 and 70 hours.
- The UK has the highest incidence of bowel cancer in the world with 20,000 new cases every year.
- Book an appointment with a colon hydrotherapist and clear your colon of obstructive waste. Once the colon is clean and efficient, detoxification and elimination will be enhanced, setting the foundation for exceptional health.
- Detoxification can bring with it symptoms of discomfort, but the process will be worth it. Through detoxification you set yourself free from the shackles of toxicity and open the gateway for a life of scintillating pleasure. Enjoy.

Be strong! Stick to your guns and prepare to embrace illuminating health with open arms. Use what you've learned and bulldoze through any negative impulses or unnatural desires and engrave positive nutritional habits into your mind. As you embrace detoxification, you'll lose weight as diseased cells, fat excretions, dead water, and other poisons rush into the bloodstream to be purged from the system. The unnatural part of you will waste away, leaving a new and vibrant you.

The cell is immortal. It is merely the fluid in which it floats that
degenerates –
Dr Alexis Carrel, French born American surgeon and biologist and
winner of the 1912 Nobel Prize.

THE RAW PERFECTION EVALUATION
Do you have a concrete understanding of detoxification?
Are you prepared to do whatever it takes to detoxify your body?
Do you continue to eat powerful raw plant foods?

CHAPTER 6

AEROBIC EXERCISE:
THE CRITICAL DAILY ROUTINE

♦ A Harvard University study, documented in the New England Journal of Medicine, followed almost 17,000 men to determine the correlation between exercise and longevity. It showed that men who walked more than nine miles per week (enough to burn off 900 calories) had a risk of death 21% lower than that of men who walked less than three miles weekly.

♦ Dr Ralph Paffenbarger of the University of California at Berkeley conducted a second long-term study of 10,000 Harvard graduates. It clearly showed that men aged between 45 and 84 who take up moderately vigorous forms of exercise (tennis, swimming, jogging, or brisk walking) reduce their overall death rates by as much as 29% and have a 41% lower risk of coronary artery disease.

♦ An eight-year study conducted by the Stanford University School of Medicine, Palo Alto, California, looked at the health habits of 10,269 Harvard University alumni over an eight-year period. The study showed that moderately active men, who took part in such sports as jogging, swimming, and running, had a 23% lower risk of dying from any cause than men who never exercised.

♦ Another study, sponsored by the Institute for Aerobics Research in Dallas, followed more than 10,000 men and 3,000 women for an average of more than eight years. They found that exercising participants in the study had lower reported rates of colon cancer, coronary heart disease, hypertension, and stroke.

♦ In a study conducted at the University of Utah Medical School, researchers found that regular participation in such activities as walking, bowling, raking leaves and ballroom dancing were enough to reduce the risk of heart attack by 30%. Another study at the University of Wisconsin Medical School showed that when heart attack patients took part in special exercise programmes, they cut their death rate from coronary artery disease by 25% – about the same rate achieved by the use of drugs, but without any toxic side effects!

♦ The benefits of exercise are so far-reaching that they even extend to organs that you wouldn't usually associate with physical fitness, such as the eyes. Exercise significantly reduces pressure against the eyeball, which causes glaucoma and frequently leads to blindness. Exercise even optimises the eyesight of people with no vision problems. A study of regular exercisers with 20/20 vision revealed that they had visual skills far superior to those sedentary people who also had 20/20 vision.

♦ But that's not all. Exercise is also a great appetite stabiliser. People with sedentary lifestyles tend to have poor appetite control and eat more than their body requires. Physical activity appears to be essential to balance appetite in line with body needs.

Need I say more! You are designed to move, remain agile and fully active until your final moments on earth! The important question is:

WHAT KIND, HOW MUCH, HOW OFTEN, AND HOW HARD?

I don't know whether or not you've been to a gym, or work out every day, maybe you consider yourself somewhere in between. One thing is for sure, there are no excuses. If you don't exercise at all, any type of exercise will increase the quality and the length of your life because movement is a critical nutrient essential for life! You are about to learn about the bare minimum, the base line standard, the level that you will always strive to stay above, whatever challenges life throws at you! If you are an athlete, the first part of this chapter isn't for you, but you might know of someone who could benefit from the following prescription. For everyone else, ask yourself the following question: What is the minimum amount of exercise necessary before reaching a point of no returns, with regard to longevity?

IF THIS ISN'T EASY ENOUGH, YOU ARE READING THE WRONG BOOK!

The following table was compiled through research taken from Harvard graduates. Treat this as your minimum daily requirement and success is yours.

Activity	Male (time in minutes)	Female (time in minutes)
Rowing	24	32
Bicycling	26	35
Swimming	26	35
Stationary bike	30	40
Jogging slowly	30	40
Walking briskly	35	47
Walking slowly	69	94

So what do these figures equate to in terms of calories? Answer: An approximate calorie expenditure of 2000 calories per week/just under 300 calories a day. If you're female, a simple 40 – 50 minute walk every day will reduce your risk of breast cancer by a staggering 70%. Amazing!

WHY WILL AEROBIC EXERCISE CHANGE YOUR LIFE?

The term 'aerobic' means, literally, 'with oxygen,' and refers to the kind of moderate exercise you can sustain over the kind of time frames given in the previous table. Your aerobic system gives you your endurance. It conditions your heart, lungs, blood vessels, and aerobic muscles and also gives you tremendous control over the hormone insulin allowing you to access your fat burning potential!

If you take long walks or jog or swim, within a matter of a few months you can restore your oxygen uptake levels similar to that of someone 20 or more years younger.

CHOOSE AEROBIC TRAINING AS A CRITICAL TOOL IN YOUR INSULIN CONTROLLING ARSENAL

By the end of RAW PERFECTION, you'll have a clear understanding of how and why you need to control the hormone insulin if you ever want to optimise your health. Insulin is your body's primary 'fat storage' hormone and if produced in excess can rob you of your health (although a certain amount must be produced to maintain optimal blood sugar levels).

Researchers at UCLA demonstrated that forty-five minutes of aerobic exercise has the same effect in lowering blood sugar levels as a single maximum injection of insulin. When you exercise, your muscles engage in continuous rhythmical contractions that draw sugar into the muscle and as sugar is utilised by the muscles, your body doesn't have to make as much insulin. Researchers at Duke University have found that by lowering blood-insulin levels, you engage the receptors on fat cells to cause fat to be released and used as energy by the body. Even after you've finished exercising and have left the gym, insulin in your body continues to operate more effectively for the next twenty-four hours.

RAW FOODISM PROPELS ATHLETES TO A WHOLE NEW LEVEL!

Overall athletic performance is sometimes determined by how efficiently a person makes use of oxygen. If your heart is well conditioned in delivering oxygenated blood to the muscles of your body, and your muscles are good at extracting that oxygen once it arrives, you'll benefit from exceptional fitness. By consistently placing the minimum demands on your body, you'll strengthen your heart, increase the number of oxygen-carrying red cells in your blood and enlarge the smaller blood vessels in your body. Gradually, through consistent conditioning, you'll also speed up the rate at which enzymes in your muscle cells utilise oxygen.

In the 1930s Professor Karl Eimer, director of the Medical Clinic at the University of Vienna, devised an excellent experiment to test the power of 100% raw-foodism on several top athletes in his country. He put them on a high-intensity physical training program for two weeks without making any alterations to their diet, then, without any transition, he placed them on a diet of 100% raw foods. Every single athlete experienced faster reflexes, more flexibility, and improved stamina.

Remember a completely raw diet will:

♦ Stimulate muscle cells to absorb nutrients and excrete waste more efficiently.
♦ Flush away the toxic residue that can develop between cells if too much refined 'junk' food has been eaten.
♦ Increase the exchange of oxygen, wastes, and nutrients at a cellular level leading to total cell efficiency.
♦ Give the muscle cells the ideal conditions to thrive and generate energy.
♦ According to Dr. Arthur Robinson, co-founder of the Linus Pauling Institute, wheatgrass juice causes your blood vessels to dilate, leading to an increase in overall blood flow, enhancing athletic performance.
♦ Many athletes have shattered personal bests with the inclusion of E3Live in their diet. Use it!

OXYGEN: THE FAT LOSS KEY

Although a well-maintained hormonal system will ensure you burn fat primarily (as you'll learn in the next two chapters), oxygen is the key for releasing it. The greater your supply of oxygen to all parts of your body, and the greater your ability to make use of it, the higher your metabolic rate, and the more success you will have in burning unwanted fat. Whenever you're inactive for extended periods of time your system doesn't eliminate toxicity as efficiently. A lack of activity also leads to poor control over blood insulin levels, leading to less appetite control.

INACTIVITY CAN LEAD TO CRAVINGS

When you are inactive, the likelihood of feeling both physically and emotionally low increases. At this point you are more inclined to reach for a chocolate bar or high fat/sugary snack. This experience has a great deal to do with the fact that neither your brain, nor the cells in the rest of your body are receiving the oxygen they need to function efficiently, giving rise to the temptation to stimulate your senses with an artificial substance. Use aerobic exercise to your advantage.

RESET YOUR BODY'S SET POINT
INCREASE YOUR METABOLIC RATE

If you've ever starved yourself in an effort to lose weight, without exercising, you've probably experienced the 'set point' phenomenon. Let me explain. Your body has an internal mechanism that regulates the amount of body fat you usually store. After a few days of reduced calorie intake, your body adjusts by lowering its basal metabolic rate (BMR), to ensure a more efficient use of the calories. This automatic biological response (the set-point phenomenon) makes it progressively difficult to lose weight whilst dieting. RAW PERFECTION promotes calorie restriction but only once you've mastered the use of nutrient dense food. Calorie restriction is the last step of mastery, certainly not the first! More about that later.

Back to the chase. How do you reset your body's set point? The answer: Exercise regularly. To date, this is the only known way to lower your set point, raise your metabolic rate, and "program" your body to store less fat than it did before. When you improve your body's use of oxygen through regular exercise, you increase your overall metabolic rate. Studies with athletes show that even 15 hours after strenuous exercise the metabolic rate is distinctly elevated, sometimes as much as 25% above normal.

MAINTAIN AN EFFICIENT METABOLISM
AND DEVELOP A SLENDER FIGURE

The measurement of how well your body is able to extract oxygen from the environment is expressed as your VO2max, or 'maximum oxygen uptake'. In most people this measurement declines steadily after the age of 30 – at a rate of about 1% a year. This decline, and the decline in overall metabolic rate that accompanies it, is a major reason why, as people get older, they get fatter! A sedentary lifestyle invites a natural decrease in your VO2 Max and encourages the deterioration of the rest of your body, skin and joints. What price do you want to pay? The small one that deals with exercise or the big one that deals with a body which has totally degenerated?

CHOOSE YOUR FUEL WISELY

Wouldn't you love to burn maximum amounts of fat when you exercise? Wouldn't you love to know that with every step you take on the treadmill, or every pull of the rowing machine, or with every peddle of the bike, you are stripping your body of unwanted fat? If you want to burn fat when you exercise, it's important you make a simple distinction. If you don't, you'll never be able to burn unlimited amounts of fat without burning out! Let me give you a clear example. Take a marathon runner for example. To complete a typical marathon, a runner will use approximately 2000 calories of energy. The question: Where does this energy come from? The two primary sources are as follows:

1. 2000 calories represents the maximum amount of carbohydrate a runner can store within their muscles and liver. This is obviously an *ineffective* source of fuel.

2. Let's now look at stored body fat as a source of fuel. A typical 150-pound marathon runner with 10% body fat, would carry 15 pounds of total fat. 3 pounds of that total fat is not accessible for energy because it's in places like the brain, and surrounding vital organs, leaving about 12 pounds of fat for possible energy use. Do you have any idea how many calories are in a pound of fat? …3500! So with a few more calculations it is easy to see that this 150-pound runner has a potential of 42000 calories of energy tucked away as fat. All they have to do to

unlock this unlimited store is eat in accordance with the principles of hormonal control and follow the advice in this chapter!

When it comes to maximising human potential in the realm of health and fitness, look no further than...

STU MITTLEMAN: WORLD RECORD HOLDER FOR RUNNING 1000 MILES IN 11 DAYS AND 19 HOURS

Stu Mittleman made it his mission to break a world record! For eleven straight days, he ran 21 hours a day and slept a mere 3 hours a night as he focused entirely on his goal. Stu demonstrated the unlimited physical potential that resides within us all. He broke the 1000-mile record by running for eleven days and nineteen hours, at an average of 84 miles per day. His demonstration was simple. Anything is possible if we make the right demands upon ourselves incrementally.

THE POWER OF ROLE MODELS

Whenever you study any area of life, always look for someone who is producing results, so you can emulate them. If you speak to anyone who witnessed the amazing 1000-mile record, they said Stu looked better at the end than he did at the beginning. He experienced no injuries, not even a blister! The distinction that he made which you'll also make is that health and fitness are not the same.

- ♦ Fitness is the physical ability to perform athletic activity.
- ♦ Health, however, is defined as the state where all the systems of the body – nervous, muscular, skeletal, circulatory, digestive, lymphatic, hormonal, etc. – are working in harmony.

Most people think that fitness implies health, but the truth is that they don't necessarily go hand in hand. It's ideal to have both health and fitness, but by putting health first, you will always enjoy tremendous benefits in your life. The optimum balance of health and fitness is achieved by training your metabolism. Remember Stu was running 84 miles a day for 11 days. Marathon runners don't even reach 30 miles!

BUILDING THE FOUNDATION OF SUCCESS

Do you want to follow in Stu's footsteps? Probably not! But do you want to apply the same principles he applied so you too can achieve amazing results? If the answer is yes, you need to realise that all exercise programs require that you begin by building an aerobic base – a period of time during which time your entire exercise program is based around aerobic activity without any anaerobic exercise at all. This base period may last from a minimum of two to a maximum of about eight months, during which your aerobic system is developed and maximised. This base period is then followed by anaerobic workouts of one, two, or sometimes three per week.

Properly developing your aerobic system will not only make you a better athlete, but it will also burn off any extra unwanted fat you may be carrying, improve your immune system, give you more energy, and keep you relatively injury-free. In other words, it's a way to build your total health and fitness through both the proper conditioning of your metabolism for aerobic and, when appropriate, anaerobic training.

DEHYDRATION – THE WORRYING HEALTH HAZARD

In 1982, Alberto Salazar won the Boston Marathon, but his celebrations were cut short when upon finishing he was immediately rushed to the emergency room at Boston Hospital where he received six litres of intravenous solution to replenish lost water and salt. Dehydration had caused him to overheat.

At an iron man race lasting between 9 and 15 hours, 64 athletes were monitored for dehydration. The study showed 27% were hyponatremic (salt deficient) and 17% of them needed medical attention. Sodium is critical. It is necessary for maintaining normal osmotic pressure and for the transport of nutrients and waste to and from cells. It also facilitates communication between cells and enables ATP generation, which is vital for energy production. The importance of sodium for athletes cannot be overstated.

Whenever you train, end your workout with a celery-based juice. Celery/apple juice and celery/kale/cucumber juice are both favourites of mine.

Remember, your body is composed of approximately 67% water. Blood is 83% water, muscles 75%, brain 75%, heart 75%, bones 22%, lungs 86%, kidneys 83%, and eyes 95%. A drop of as little as 2% will cause tiredness and fatigue. A 10% drop can cause significant health problems.

ARE YOU READY FOR THE CHALLENGE?
THE ADVANCED AEROBIC PRESCRIPTION

Your goal is to burn more fat than carbohydrates during exercise. If however, you begin exercising too hard the process that involves the transportation of fat from adipose tissue to your muscles is often compromised. By controlling the two master hormones of energy metabolism (insulin and glucagon) you can get a greater control over this process. More about this in chapter 11 – Exercise: The Champion Hormonal Regulator. For now realise that you want to steer away from burning stored carbohydrate within the muscle. You want to burn fat. This is easily done if you follow this prescription and write your heart rates in the spaces provided:

1. BUY A HEART RATE MONITOR TODAY!
2. Work out your maximum heart rate.
   220 minus your age = maximum heart rate....................Never exceed this.
3. Using your maximum heart rate work out your warm up and cool down rate.

Aerobic Warm up and Cool-down
Max Heart rate x 60% = warm up (high end).......................
Max Heart rate x 55% = warm up (low end).......................

If you warm up for 15 minutes at this low intensity you mobilise any free fatty acids stored within your body. Fat will then get used as your primary fuel instead of stored carbohydrate. In this period of time, you give your body the time to gradually distribute blood to the areas that need it, rather than immediately shunting it away from vital organs. And that is all it takes. By controlling insulin and glucagon levels and preventing low blood sugar levels, you'll find yourself working out and feeling great. More about this in the next chapter.

4. Once you've completed your warm-up, exercise within your aerobic training zone for between 20 and 45 minutes. Use the following formula to work out your heart rate range.

Optimal Aerobic Training Zone
180 minus your age = ...
This is your maximum aerobic heart rate during training before your body switches to anaerobic metabolism.
Take this figure and subtract 10 points, then keep your heart rate between these two figures.
Write the two figures here................. - .... This will be your optimal aerobic training zone.

Other points to remember are as follows:
- If you are recovering from a major illness or are on medication subtract an additional 10 points
- If you have not exercised before, have an injury, are gearing down in your training, or if you often get colds or flu, or have allergies subtract 5 points.
- If you have been exercising for up to two years without any real problems, and have not had colds or flu more than once or twice a year, keep your score the same.
- If you have been exercising for more than two years without any problems, while making progress in competition without injury, add 5 points.

5. Finally, remember to cool down for 15 minutes after your main exercise routine before you stretch. By cooling down, you'll prevent blood from pooling in your working muscles. When people stop exercising suddenly, it's difficult for the blood to be returned for cleansing, re-oxygenation and redistribution. Stretching is also recommended. Whether you engage in a simple stretch program or prefer to practice Yoga or Pilates, a diet high in green leafy vegetables will create a more alkaline environment in your body and free up your range of movement.

TIME: A PERSONAL PREFERENCE

Whatever time of day you choose to exercise is entirely your decision. You may only be able to fit exercise into a certain part of your day and have to stick to it. If you have the flexibility to try different routines then this will give you the chance to find out what works for you. The best all round day begins with stretching to mobilise the body (I recommend The Egoscue Method. Go to www.egoscue.com and take a look for yourself), however you can continue your routine by completing all your other exercises. If you train in the morning, you'll feel an unprecedented explosion of energy that will linger throughout the day, helping you to steer away from food and caffeine to wake you up. If you choose to train in the afternoon, you'll be rewarding your body and mind with a natural injection of endorphins. If you find that you like to work well into the night, then ensure you have a mild evening workout. The extra oxygen and movement will wake your body up and allow you to burn the midnight oil. You'll learn about the power of resistance training in chapter 11 – Exercise – The Champion Hormonal Regulator, but for now if you love training with weights you need to understand the power of…

TESTOSTERONE:
HORMONE OF STRENGTH, POWER AND DESIRE

The production of testosterone is under circadian rhythm control. It peaks in the morning, and then falls during the day. The highest levels occur between 2am and 4am and stay elevated until about 9am, making the morning a better time to train with weights. Bill Pearl (four times Mr Universe Bodybuilding champion and the only man to defeat Arnold Schwarzenegger for the Mr Universe title) always did his training at 3am in order to utilise the maximum release of testosterone. By 3pm, testosterone levels will have dropped by some 40% compared to the morning. It's also worth noting that Bill Pearl is a strict vegetarian.

THE RAW PERFECTION EVALUATION:
Do you engage in aerobic exercise to build unshakeable health?
Are you following the advanced aerobic prescription?

PART TWO

FINE-TUNING THE HORMONAL PHILHARMONIC

You've created the foundation for optimal health. Now it's time to fine tune your knowledge and step up the pace! Prepare to...

CHAPTER 7

KICKSTART YOUR FAT METABOLISM: TAMING THE INSULIN DRAGON

Many people want to lose weight and many people are on diets, but how many people do you see fail in their quest for a slim body time after time? If you want the struggle to come to a grinding halt you MUST learn to control...

THE HORMONE PHILHARMONIC

The hormones of your body are like the musicians of an orchestra playing a beautiful symphony. When the orchestra is playing in tune, the symphony sounds wonderful. If, however one of the musicians plays too loudly, or is out of sync with the others, the symphony can sound horrific. In your body, if one hormone begins to predominate it can cause devastating effects and suppress the action of other hormones. In today's society, it is easy to engage in habits that over-stimulate the hormone insulin. An excess of which can lead to weight gain and cause utter chaos within the body. It's up to you to use food correctly and thus maintain tight control of the hormone philharmonic, securing an abundance of health and vitality.

INSULIN: CRITICAL TO HEALTH
YET POTENTIALLY LIFE THREATENING

As you read RAW PERFECTION, you'll see that insulin gets a hard time. I even go as far labelling insulin as the enemy! The truth is – if insulin didn't get released from your pancreas to control the level of sugar in your bloodstream, your health would deteriorate rapidly and you'd die! If your central nervous system detects a rising in blood sugar levels, it is considered a life-threatening danger and signals are sent to the various sites in the body to release the hormones necessary to restore those levels. Normal blood sugar levels are approximately 60mg/dl to 120mg/dl (mg/dl = milligrams of glucose in 100 millilitres of blood), and very high levels, such as 800mg/dl, can lead to coma and death. Insulin prevents blood sugar levels from rising too high, making it an important part of your hormonal balancing act – but at the same time…

INSULIN IS 30 TIMES MORE EFFECTIVE AT SHUNTING
EXTRA CALORIES INTO *FAT* THAN INTO *MUSCLE*

The goal of this chapter is to direct the flow of fat away from fat tissue and towards the muscles to be burnt for energy, and the only way to do this is to learn how to minimise insulin production within your body. If insulin is 30 times more effective at shunting extra calories into fat than into muscle, you need to take some effective action. All you need to remember is that most hormones work together as part of a balancing act. Most people over-stimulate insulin and under-stimulate it's partner glucagon, leading to imbalance. By learning what foods stimulate insulin you can reduce their consumption, and by learning how to stimulate glucagon you can restore hormonal balance. If glucagon predominates you'll have tuned into the fat burning pathway, burning up excess fat whilst you speed down the road towards a slim, healthy, vibrant body, singing and dancing all the way! Remember, insulin makes you fat and keeps you fat and glucagons makes you thin and keeps you thin. Let me now introduce you to the term 'Benign Dietary Ketosis' (BDK), because it is a magical method for kick-starting your fat metabolism…

WHY IS THERE SO MUCH MAGIC IN THIS METHOD?

The term ketosis is really a shortening of the term ketosis/lipolysis and if you want to dissolve fat then this is certainly the way forward. The definition of lipolysis is simple. It means nothing less than the dissolving of fat. Fat gets broken down into glycerol and free-fatty acids. The fatty acids then break down into ketone bodies (which can be used as fuel) and a shorter fatty acid. Apart from being a storage site for poisonous wastes and toxins, fat is nothing but stored energy. The key to storing this energy is the hormone insulin. If you want to pile on the pounds, insulin is your most valuable asset, it safely tucks fat away in the places you hate to see it, around your belly, on your hips and at the tops of your legs etc., and it also prevents the burning of fat – That is why it is critical to eliminate foods that over-stimulate it.

When you kickstart your fat burning metabolism you'll enter the fat-dissolving state known as BDK, or ketosis/lipolysis. This fat-dissolving state can only be accessed by minimising insulin secretion. Remember, if your body can easily become a fat storage machine, it can also become a fat burning machine. If people can gain weight easily, science says there should be a method for stripping the body of fat as easily. This is where you are headed. Fat will be your primary fuel, so get ready for some serious fat loss as you safely release ketones and utilise the metabolic pathway that is the complete opposite to that which got you fat in the first place.

KETOSIS/LIPOLYSIS IS YOUR ANSWER TO BURNING FAT BUT WHAT ABOUT CALORIES?

If you've spent your life trying to lose weight, you've probably spent a lifetime worrying about calories. Let me tell you, calories should be the least of your concerns. Traditional calorie thinking says,

"A calorie is a calorie and that is all that matters. A gram of fat has more than twice the calories of a gram of carbohydrate, so you can eat twice as much carbohydrate as fat and you'll lose weight"

Wrong! The key to understanding fat loss, is understanding the effect food has on your hormonal response. To think hormonally would be to think that a calorie of fat has a different hormonal effect than a calorie of carbohydrate, and a calorie of protein has a different effect still.

IT'S NOT ABOUT CALORIES
IT'S ABOUT HORMONAL CONTROL

I'll repeat. IT'S NOT ABOUT CALORIES! IT'S ABOUT HORMONAL CONTROL! If you've spent your whole life focusing exclusively on calories – STOP! Your hormonal response to food is the only factor you need to be concerned with! For some of you this won't be easy to digest because you've been following the low calorie mindset for so many years. There is nothing wrong with lowering calorie intake, but the most important factor is controlling what foods make up these calories. Let me present you with some information about a classic study done over forty years ago.

TAKE CONTROL OF MACRO-NUTRIENT RATIOS
AND PREPARE FOR SOME SERIOUS WEIGHT LOSS

In the early part of the 1950s, Professor Alan Kekwick, Director of the Institute of Clinical Research and Experimental Medicine at London's prestigious Middlesex Hospital, and Dr Gaston L.S. Pawan, Senior Research Biochemist of the hospital's medical unit embarked on a fascinating journey into the world of macro-nutrient ratios.

Their wonderful journey began when they became intrigued with various studies that suggested that weight loss was controlled by varying the macro-nutrient content of the diet (i.e. changing fat, protein and carbohydrate ratios). Their fascination was sparked by the clinical studies of Dr. Alfred W Pennington on employees of the Dupont Corporation along with German and Scandinavian papers showing success with diet plans that had very restricted carbohydrate quantities.

They decided to conduct their own experiments on a group of obese subjects to test the results for themselves:
♦ Those on a 90% protein intake lost weight.
♦ Those on a 90% fat intake lost weight.
♦ But when subjects were given a diet of which 90% of the calories came from carbohydrates, they didn't lose a pound.

Note: If you restrict calories to the extreme, weight loss may occur but at the expense of high quality nutrition. Weight lost by this method of dieting is usually water and muscle wastage.

Back to the chase. The tests performed by Kekwick and Pawan were simple, but they were both so overwhelmed by the results, they devoted nearly 20 years to researching why calories seemed to be of no importance in dieting!

SEPARATE YOURSELF FROM THE MASSES AND WAVE GOODBYE TO FAILURE!

In their preliminary studies Kekwick and Pawan found that a diet of 1000 calories per week was only successful when most of the calories came from fat and protein, yet a carbohydrate diet consisting of 1000 calories per week produced very little weight loss. This proved that it's not the calories alone that make the difference but the foods that make up those calories. With this in mind, it is easy to see why there are such diverse results within weight loss groups. Everyone can adhere to a low calorie diet, but individual food choices will always be different. If the process of weight loss was simply a matter of controlling calorie intake, then regardless of what foods the calories came from, everyone would experience similar results. This certainly isn't the case!

MELT FAT OFF OF YOUR BODY AND ELIMINATE UNUSED CALORIES

Kekwick and Pawan found that even on a balanced 2000-calorie diet, subjects experienced no fat loss. Yet when their diet was mainly fat, these same obese subjects could lose unwanted body fat even when consuming 2600 calories. Being uniquely thorough, Kekwick and Pawan did water balance studies proving that the weight being lost was mostly fat.

BRING ON THE MICE AND THE METABOLIC CHAMBER!

Next, they embarked on a study of mice in a metabolic chamber. They measured the loss of carbon in their excretions and were able to show that on the high fat diet, mice excreted considerable quantities of unused calories in the form of ketone bodies. At the end of the study period, they analysed the fat content of the animals' bodies and found significant decreases in percentage body fat.

THE MAGIC AND MYSTERY OF
THE FAT MOBILISATION SUBSTANCE

During their wonderful adventure, Kekwick and Pawan discovered and extracted a substance from the urine of the low-carbohydrate dieters. When this substance was injected into non-dieting animals and humans it caused them to experience rapid weight loss, a massive decrease in the percentage of carcass fat, an increase in ketone and free fatty-acid levels and an increase in the excretion of unused calories from 10% to 36%!

The substance they stumbled over was a Fat Mobilisation Substance (FMS) and as researchers discovered other substances that effected metabolism in the same way, they labelled them lipid mobilisers. These lipid mobilisers are your primary weapon for kick-starting fat loss as they enables you to excrete unused calories that may have been stored in your body on the low fat-high carbohydrate diet. If you need any more evidence...

HIBERNATING ANIMALS PROVE
THERE IS ONLY ONE WAY: NATURES WAY

In the absence of carbohydrate, your body sends out a signal to release a generous influx of lipid mobilisers. If you look into nature, the burning of stored fat in the absence of dietary carbohydrate is what sustains hibernating animals. The intelligence and wisdom of your body provides a variety of natural messenger substances to ensure that fat mobilisation is efficient and quick. This is the state any obese person should be striving for and represents the road to success! The immediate feedback is great; i.e. the pounds drop off at an amazing rate and energy levels soar.

SO MANY STUDIES, SO MANY RESULTS

Frederick Benoit and his associates at the Oakland Naval Hospital decided to compare two methods of losing weight with seven men weighing between 230 and 290 pounds. The methods are as follows:

1. A 1000-calorie diet, with 10 gram carbohydrate and high fat.
2. Fasting
♦ The first method saw the men lose 14.5 pounds, and out of this 14 pounds was body fat.
♦ On the 10 day fast, the men lost 21 pounds on average, but most of that was lean body weight. Only 7.5 pounds was body fat.

Benoit's other exciting discovery was that on the ketogenic diet, the dieters maintained adequate potassium levels, whilst the second group lost severe amounts of potassium. About a decade later, many dieters lost their lives on very low calorie diets similar to fasting. Many individuals hypothesised that the deaths were due to potassium losses, leading to heart arrhythmia, but there is another theory that if too much toxicity is allowed to enter the bloodstream too quickly (in the case of obese subjects), it can suffocate the individual. In the case of rapid weight loss, natural measures must be used to keep the blood thin and clean, and exercise/stretching must be used as it enhances the healing process. Go back to chapter 5 - Detoxification to re-cap.

MAXIMISE YOUR FAT BURNING POTENTIAL

Charlotte Young, professor of Clinical Nutrition at Cornell University published an interesting study. She chose overweight young men as her subjects, and put them on various diets. Each of the three diets was based around carbohydrate restriction and consisted of 1800 calories. The results were recorded for nine weeks.

♦ Diet 1 contained 104 grams of carbohydrate and the subjects lost 2.73 pounds per week, of which 2 pounds was body fat.
♦ Diet 2 contained 60 grams of carbohydrate and subjects lost 3 pounds per week, of which 2.5 pounds was body fat.
♦ Diet 3 contained 30 grams of carbohydrate and the subjects lost 3.73 pounds per week, all of which was body fat. This group was producing ketosis and FMS.

By dropping 74 grams of insulin inducing carbohydrate and replacing it with 300 calories of glucagon stimulating protein based food, these young men lost an extra 1.7 pounds of body fat each and every week.

INSULIN: A SAVIOUR AND SILENT KILLER
THE EFFECT OF FOOD COMBINATIONS
ON INSULIN AND GLUCAGON

Through scientific investigation, subjects had their blood taken and analysed after many different food combinations to determine how much impact the food had on the two hormones of energy metabolism; insulin and glucagon. The results are as follows.

FOOD COMBINATION	INSULIN	GLUCAGON
Carbohydrate	+++++	No change
Protein	++	++
Fat	No change	No change
Carbohydrate and Fat	++++	No change
Protein and Fat	++	++
High Protein and Low Carbohydrate	++	+
High Carbohydrate and Low Protein	+++++++++	+

AVOID THE 'BEST-SELLERS' PROMOTING MEAT TO
STIMULATE GLUCAGON

Many national best-selling books on nutrition will teach you that in order to minimise insulin production and thus avoid aggressive fat storage, you need to stimulate the hormone glucagon and eliminate refined carbohydrates. This information is correct, however many of them suggest eating meat to stimulate glucagon. They say that whenever you're hungry you can eat steak, eggs, fish or certain cheeses and lose more body fat than ever before! This may come as exciting news to you if you love meat, but there is a downside. Toxicity!

The other problem is that of 'vegetarianism'. Most vegetarians eliminate meat in order to improve health and become addicted to pasta, rice and baked potatoes, all of which are high in carbohydrate, stimulate insulin and supply minimal nutrition. Cheese is another favourite food for vegetarians but is high in saturated fat, is very mucus forming and supplies minimal nutrition. A better strategy for long term health is to eliminate refined carbohydrates and eat a diet of green plant foods, raw plant fats, vegetables and fruit. Although meat stimulates glucagon, it does so at the expense of adding toxicity to your body. The pay off isn't worth it in the end. A better strategy would be to use soy. Soy stimulates insulin less than meat and has more of a stimulating effect on glucagon. Think of Soy as your no.1 fat loss food along with green leafy vegetables and raw plant fats.

NATURES SUPER-PROTEIN –
EXPAND YOUR AWARENESS OF SOY

♦ In countries where soy products are eaten regularly, rates of heart disease are low. Consumption of soy products causes a decrease in both total cholesterol and LDL cholesterol levels.
♦ In Asian countries where diets are rich in soy, rates of breast cancer are much lower. Japanese women have only one-quarter the rate of breast cancer of American women.
♦ Japanese males (who consume a lot of soy) have far lower rates of prostate cancer than their counterparts in America.
♦ Researchers have found that compounds in soy foods (isoflavones) help to ease the symptoms of menopause such as night sweats and hot flushes. In some cases by 40%. Isoflavones can act as oestrogens, which help to compensate for decreased natural oestrogen production during menopause.
♦ The high calcium content of soy rich foods can decrease rates of bone loss and increase bone density.

PREVENT CANCER WITH THE POWER OF SOY
AND AVOID THE PERILS OF MEATS

German scientists isolated an enzyme in the urine of people who eat a Japanese diet heavy in soybeans and vegetables. They then used that enzyme (also found in cruciferous vegetables, such as cabbage) in test-tube experiments, and found that it can block the growth of new blood vessels that feed malignant tumours, preventing them from growing, invading the blood/lymph systems, and spreading throughout the body.

Cytologists have carried out an immense amount of research in order to discover differences between the structures of normal cells and those of cancer cells. They have found that cancer cells are of a basic structure, lacking useful capability and differentiation. Their only purpose is to devour dead proteins (typically of animal origin) and multiply.

WAR PROVIDES VALUABLE INSIGHTS INTO THE PERILS OF COOKED FOODS AND MEAT

Considerable evidence has been collected by research scientists all over the world showing that when cooked foods are eliminated, so is the incidence and growth of cancer. During the Gotterdammerung (the two world wars) under severe food rationing in Austria, Germany, Russia, Britain, and Poland, cancer deaths declined dramatically.

When the Germans occupied Norway during the Second World War, the Norwegian government was forced to sharply reduce the availability of dead animals to its citizens. Of course, the death rate from cancer and circulatory diseases plummeted. After the war, the Norwegians returned to their former diet and the death rates rose again as before. Among wild animals in nature, cancer is unknown. However, after subjecting captive monkeys to degenerated foods for extended periods of time, cancer begins to appear. Only those animals that have not reached the cooked hands of humanity are safe.

During the Vietnam War, some American POWs were condemned to death by being fed a diet consisting exclusively of cooked meat. Many did not survive longer than one month, whereas in the event of complete fasting, a person may survive as long as one hundred days. This clearly demonstrates that not only is cooked meat a degenerative foodstuff, but a poison that has the potential to kill its victim.

YOUR ULTIMATE SOURCE OF PROTEIN – E3LIVE AFA ALGAE

E3Live is an exceptionally high source of quality protein (60%) and is superior to that of most other plant or animal protein sources. If you are vegetarian and don't eat an abundance of green leafy vegetables combined with raw plant fats, you may tend to suffer from a deficiency of basic protein. Fish, chicken, beef, turkey, etc. may contain all eight essential amino acids to form complete protein, but your body finds them difficult to digest. When protein digestion is incomplete, bacteria can form toxic compounds. However, the protein found in AFA algae, is a type called glycoprotein. Meat and vegetable protein is of a type called lipoprotein. The body has to convert lipoproteins into glycoproteins in order to utilise them, and in the process digestive energies are used up. On the other hand AFA algae protein is more biochemically efficient and 85% assimilable. Beef however has just a 20% assimilable. Eliminate meat and begin the daily intake of E3Live. Incomplete protein digestion produces toxins, and may render the protein worthless anyway.

ENHANCE HORMONAL CONTROL – CLEAN OUT YOUR COLON

Towards the middle of the pancreas there is a group of glands of internal secretion, known as the islands of langerhans, which produce insulin. In a toxic body where the colon is afflicted with fermentation and putrefaction, the islands of langerhans are thwarted from producing optimal amounts of insulin necessary to control blood sugar levels. Ironically, the foods that cause toxicity also stimulate aggressive insulin secretion. This helps to highlight why so many people suffer with adult onset Type II diabetes, and sometimes have to begin injecting insulin. The first step to recovery is by cleansing the colon with a series of colon irrigations. If this can be backed up with the principles of RAW PERFECTION, complete recovery can be made, and insulin injections avoided.

GEAR YOUR BODY TOWARDS WEIGHT LOSS ESCAPE THE TRAP AND LOSE A POUND OF BODY FAT EVERY OTHER DAY!

If you are overweight and have been for some time, you probably feel trapped. High insulin levels have kept you trapped, but the kick-start principle can set you free allowing you to lose up to a pound of body fat every other day! I used to be taught that you could only lose 1-2 pounds per week – Maximum! Think about it, if some people can put on 14 pounds of unwanted fat in a few short weeks, then the body must have a mechanism to shed body fat that quickly as well – it makes sense. And by using the principle of Benign Dietary Ketosis (BDK) you have at your finger tips a major weapon, and it's powerful enough to win the war single handily against obesity. In order to melt fat from your body once and for all, you need to remember a few important lessons:

1. Firstly, the over-production of insulin is the reason you have become fat and stayed fat.

♦ Recreational foods are full of sugar and over-stimulate insulin. Eliminate them!

Too many people spend all day nibbling! A biscuit here, a chocolate bar there, a packet of crisps etc. Each of these foods but keep insulin levels elevated adding to the ongoing problem of obesity. Eliminate them!

♦ Recreational foods are full of saturated cooked fats and increase insulin levels.

Saturated fat promotes a higher glucose load in the blood and interferes with the membranes of your cells. The result: Insulin sensors malfunction and your body pumps out more insulin to bring blood sugar levels down. Combine saturated cooked fats with the high glucose load of cooked carbohydrates and you unleash the biggest hormonal nightmare of all. Studies have shown that if rats are fed a diet with a macronutrient ratio equal to 40% cooked fat and 40% sugar, fat storage levels increased more than any other combination of foods. We are talking about some seriously hefty rats! If you are overweight, but don't think you eat that much, take a look at the macronutrient ratio's of your diet. Are you eating small amounts of recreational food throughout the day? Even a few biscuits or the occasional chocolate bar/cake will keep your insulin levels elevated, and promote fat storage. Saturated fat and sugar form the basis of the junk foods that occupy the supermarket shelves. Eliminate them!

PERFORM LIKE A WORLD CLASS ATHLETE: ELIMINATE SATURATED FATS

If you are serious about exercise and fitness, you'll be interested to know that saturated fats change the outer layer (membrane) of your muscle, preventing the flow of nutrients and glucose to muscle cells, compromising performance. Eliminate them!

♦ Consuming too many calories causes the over-production of insulin. Eat little and often!

If you think that *only* fat makes you fat, you are wrong! Any excess, whether it's carbohydrate, protein or fat, can end up being stored as unnecessary fat in the liver, heart, arteries, fat tissues, kidneys or muscle.

Think back to the last time you feasted. By eating too much food and overloading your body with excess calories, your body, in its infinite wisdom, releases copious amounts of insulin and stores the excess as fat for a future famine. For many people in industrialised nations, every day is a feast. Make sure you are not one of them!

THE UNLIMITED DUMPING GROUND
FOR EXCESS CALORIES

The unhappy ending to this story is that you can store unlimited amounts of fat, and insulin is the key. The excess fat deposits lay the foundation for diseases associated with fatty degeneration such as atherosclerosis, liver and kidney degeneration, tumours, obesity, rheumatic diseases and diabetes. Saturated and monounsaturated fatty acids increase tissue anoxia (lack of oxygen), choking the body's tissues. It's your choice. Advertisers lead you to believe that if a food is 99% fat free you'll stay slim. Wrong! Most of these foods are loaded with sugar. Sugar stimulates excessive amounts of insulin, putting your body into a fat storage mode. If you eat any extra cooked fat, whilst devouring carbohydrate foods, you might as well write your own obesity prescription. The equation is simple. Learn it, remember it and share it with others. Excess glucose = Excessive Insulin Secretion = Excess Fat Storage.

2. Secondly, insulin's partner glucagon causes fat-loss and is your primary fat burning weapon.

♦ <u>Stimulate glucagon and access the fat-burning pathway with protein.</u>
Some authorities suggest fish, poultry, red meat, and eggs/dairy. I used to! All these foods however cause toxicity in your body. If you want to get maximum control over your insulin levels, use soy. It has the advantage of causing less insulin secretion than animal protein, whilst stimulating more glucagon – a truly advantageous one-two punch in your favour! If you choose soy products, sprouted soybeans are an excellent choice and an excellent raw food.

♦ <u>The over-consumption of meat protein can cause unnecessary toxicity. Only eat a small portion at any one meal.</u>
If you choose to continue one 'cooked food' whilst you strip maximum fat from your body. I suggest in this order, cooked soy, fresh fish, foul,

eggs and finally red meat. I think there's more danger becoming
vegetarian and relying on high carbohydrate foods (pasta, rice, potatoes,
bread), than eliminating them and relying on small portions of meat to
accompany an abundance of green leafy vegetable, raw plant fats and
fruits. Remember, meat protein stimulates the hormone glucagon. *Your
body only utilises a small amount of protein at any one time, so ensure
you eat no more than you can fit in the palm of your hand.* This way
you'll minimise any chance of protein toxicity and maximise protein
absorption. Excess protein can also disrupt the acid/alkaline balance of
your body, so accompany your meat dish with a plentiful supply of raw
plant foods/vegetables.

♦ Eat foods that prevent excessive insulin secretion. Insulin inhibits
   glucagon.
The rate and speed that the carbohydrate gets absorbed into the blood
stream controls the rate of insulin secretion. By slowing down the rate at
which carbohydrate enters your bloodstream you can begin to control
insulin secretion and therefore control your own fat storage/burning
mechanism. Concentrate on carbohydrate sources such as fruits,
vegetables and sprouts, all of which prevent excessive insulin secretion.

ELIMINATE THE POWERFUL BONE DESTROYER

In his book "Nutrition and Physical Degeneration" by Weston Price,
D.D.S. he tells the stories of his travels around the world. He found that
when native people started eating refined flour products, it destroyed
their bones in one generation. No matter what the race of natives, the
results were consistent. Refined flour products transformed broad skulls,
wide dental arches and beautiful bodies into deformed narrow skulls
(like many if not most Western civilisations), narrow dental arches, and
misshapen bodies. White flour products, including pasta and bread, are
the worst destroyers of bone in anyone's diet. Any food that contains
refined flour is a bone poison.

DESTROYING SEXUALITY WITH BREAD

Bread is the first food you should eliminate from your diet if you want to
build any kind of health, strength or vitality. Bread contains an
enormous amount of oestrogen (a female hormone) that upsets the

natural balance of sexual hormones in men. The more bread you eat, the more likely your sexuality will suffer! Do you want male breast development or sexual dysfunction? I think not! Stack the odds in your favour by not eating it.

3. Thirdly, when you've reached your ideal weight you'll want to keep insulin and glucagon balanced.

With the right foods you can change your body from a fat-sucking machine to a fat burning machine. That is the only goal of this chapter! All you need to do is eat the foods that cause the kick-start principle to begin and simultaneously avoid the foods that cause you to retain and increase fat storage. Do this and you'll melt away fat faster than ice cream melts on a summers day. The ultimate question: Do you want to be permanently slim or temporarily slim? Do you want to have permanently high energy levels or temporary levels of energy? Temporary measures bring about temporary results.

PERMANENT MEASURES LEAD TO PERMANENT RESULTS

In the UK alone, over £25million is spent on weight loss products every year and the figure is rising. What do you think the success rate is? Are you ready for this remarkably high figure? 5%. That's right, I'll even type it out – five percent. How would you describe a 95% failure rate? I'd describe it as an absolute rip-off. Very few approaches to nutrition take into consideration the biochemical factors that cause obesity in the first place. If these diets really did work, would there be an unending chain of new ones? If diets worked, wouldn't the rate of obesity in this country be decreasing instead of increasing? Dieting has been labelled a national epidemic. It is even harder to treat than the vast majority of cancers because many so-called health practitioners are using the wrong approach, time after time!

A VICTORY IS A VICTORY WHEREVER YOU SCORE FROM ON THE PLAYING FIELD

Millions of people have lost weight and kept it off through a variety of methods. Some people kept their eating habits the same and simply introduced exercise into their daily routine. Exercise helps control insulin levels. Other people did nothing but give up chocolate and sweets, again eliminating the foods that cause excessive insulin production. High carbohydrate diets have probably worked for some people dealt the lucky cards of a fast metabolism, but even these people may have elevated insulin levels and suffer with high blood pressure regardless of their slender figure, I used to! You are probably beginning to see that there isn't a magic bullet ultimately, but there is an ultimate goal. That is to keep insulin under control.

THE MAGIC OF MINIATURE MEALS

Today you can begin to use a simple principle that will give you immediate control over your insulin levels regardless of what you eat. This principle will have an enormous impact on your body and will serve you for the rest of your life. The simple answer for all you 'wanna be slim' people out there is to forget about three square meals a day, and concentrate on smaller, more frequent eating. By fostering this approach, 'fasting morning insulin levels' drop by 25-30% allowing you to begin losing weight without even dieting.

A leading researcher in this area is Professor David Jenkins. In his classic study, entitled Nibbling versus Gorging, he discovered that in order to lower cholesterol, all you had to do was eat your normal intake of food but spread it more evenly throughout the day. If you use this advice and increase your intake of raw fruits, vegetables, sprouts and their juices, not to mention wheatgrass juice and E3Live, can you imagine the effects? Holding onto excess fat will be impossible!

THE AWESOME POWER OF GRAZING

If the grazing rather than gauging mentality causes such improvements in hormonal control, how extreme can you take this nibbling principle? A study was conducted where a number of men were split into two groups. The first ate their total food intake in three square meals, breakfast, lunch and dinner. The second group ate the same quantity of food but it was divided into 17 snacks.

The result: Group one experienced minimal changes, but group two decreased their serum insulin level by 27.9% and the key stress hormone, cortisol, by 17.3%. Controlling cortisol output is as important to RAW PERFECTION as any other principle. You'll learn more about this in chapter 11 – Eliminate Stress.

Grazing on quality food is one thing, eating anything that dares cross your path is another. Even though grazing has been proven to be an effective strategy to keep insulin, cortisol and other age related hormones under tight control, eating the wrong foods will only promote the rapid increase in unwanted body fat. Spending your whole day nibbling on refined 'recreational foods' will accelerate the ageing process and take you one step closer to an early grave. Take a look why:

♦ Low fat recreational foods are pumped full of sugar, causing insulin to spike.
♦ They are pumped full of additives and preservatives, causing you to store excess toxicity.
♦ Being processed, they deliver no 'life-force' in the way of vitamins, minerals, enzymes or phytochemicals.
♦ They leave your body nutritionally starved, which causes you to feel hungry again when you've only just eaten.
♦ Eventually they cause you to feel tired, lifeless and dead!

A RECAP: THE ROLES OF INSULIN AND GLUCAGON

INSULIN	GLUCAGON
Lowers elevated blood sugar	Raises low blood sugar
Shifts metabolism so storing fuel predominates	Shifts metabolism into a fat burning mode
Converts glucose and protein to fat	Converts protein and fat to glucose
Converts dietary fat into a form for storage	Converts dietary fats to ketones and sends them to the tissues for energy
Takes fat from the blood and transports it into cells	Releases fat from fat cells into the blood for use by tissues as energy
Increases the body's production of cholesterol	Decreases the body's production of cholesterol
Makes the kidneys retain excess fluid	Makes the kidneys release excess fluid
Stimulates the growth of arterial smooth muscle	Stimulates the regression of arterial smooth muscle
Stimulates the use of glucose for energy	Stimulates the use of fat for energy

Fortunately, for every health hazard that excess insulin causes, glucagon can reverse. Glucagon encourages the kidneys to release excess salt and fluid, ease the production of cholesterol in the liver, slow down triglyceride production, relax artery walls causing blood pressure to decline, and cause the fat cells to mobilise stored fats for energy. If insulin is produced in excess, glucagon is overwhelmed.

A NEW PIECE TO THE FASCINATING PUZZLE

Although it's critical to eliminate refined carbohydrates and refined sugar, there are some vegetables and fruits, which can also cause problems within the body if not monitored carefully. These specific fruits and vegetables are obviously healthier than their cooked food counterparts but can still jeopardise your progress. Ironically they are the plant foods many people are addicted to because of their high sugar content. Let me introduce you to hybrid food...

USING HYBRID FOODS TO YOUR ADVANTAGE

In a world where the mass production of fruits and vegetables has been a number one priority, crops have been cultivated and crossbred for a more appealing taste and longer durability. Over time they have grown genetically weaker regardless of their sweet flavours and durability. The protective human environments have forced the crops and fruit trees to adapt so much that they've lost their 'genetic energy' and are unable to survive in the wild.

WHAT'S THE BIG DEAL WITH HYBRIDISED FOODS?

Refined and processed carbohydrates must be avoided if you want to experience the joys of vibrant health, but natural sugars from hybridised foods also upset the delicate hormonal balancing act within your body. The reason behind this is that the liver doesn't recognise these sugars and they pass directly into the bloodstream causing the familiar sugar 'high' associated with sweets, and recreational 'junk' food. For example, I used to be addicted to carrot juice! Now remember, although carrot/apple or carrot/beet/celery juice has been used to cure people of some of the most debilitating illnesses (read Jay Kordich's story in his book entitled, The Juiceman), once the healing has taken place, hybridised foods should be minimised. Alternatively, other juices can be used in the place of carrot juice. Greens are an excellent base for all juices. Apples and pears are great sweeteners, and celery is an all-round superstar because of its alkaline qualities. Cucumber is also great to neutralise the bitterness of vegetables.

Hybridised foods, eaten in excess, can cause the same problems associated with the high carbohydrate, low fat diet, namely – increased insulin production, weight gain and possibly hyperinsulinemia. The first signs are extreme tiredness and fatigue! Be warned!

Hybrid foods are also low in trace nutrients, failing to satisfy the demands of your body. You may *feel* full, but you body isn't *nutritionally* full. The answer: Eat high-quality green-leafy vegetables, which have necessary trace elements, and use raw plant fats to slow down the rate in which the sugars enter the blood. Too much sugar in the blood strips away the alkaline minerals from your bones and tissues in an effort to neutralise the acidifying effects of too much sugar.

WHERE TO PLACE YOUR ATTENTION

Here's a guideline to help you minimise hybrid food:

♦ Minimise all seedless fruits or fruits with non-viable seeds; they are genetically altered and weak. These include seedless apples, bananas, several date varieties (especially medjools), kiwis, seedless pineapples, seedless citrus fruits, seedless grapes (raisins), seedless persimmons, and seedless watermelons. All the above are loaded with hybrid sugar and will upset the delicate endocrine balancing act if eaten in excess.

♦ Most people, who don't like fruit, like bananas. Bananas are excessively hybridised foods and as well as having an unnaturally high sugar content, also have unbalanced mineral ratios. Too much hybridised sweet fruit can lead to mineral deficiencies, don't eliminate them, but minimise their use.

♦ Limit the overeating/juicing of hybrid vegetables: beets, carrots, corn, and potatoes.

♦ The same rule applies for hybrid nuts and seeds: cashews, oats, rice, and wheat.

♦ As you develop more of a love for fruits and vegetables, don't discard hybrid foods indefinitely, just be aware of their potential to upset your health if eaten in excess. Awareness is the key to set you free!

♦ Always use greens and raw plant fats to dampen the effect of hybridised foods when you eat them. Examples may be bananas with nuts, avocados with hybrid fruit or vegetables, by doing so you'll decrease the release of sugars into the bloodstream.

Cooked food has a tremendously destabilising effect on blood sugar levels. When you eat cooked food you can expect blood sugar level fluctuations ten times greater than when you eat live or enzyme rich foods. Enzyme rich raw food causes a much steadier metabolic rate and greater emotional stability.

IT'S TIME FOR SOME SIMPLE SACRIFICES

For you to get the maximum out of the Kick-start Principle there are certain boundaries and rules, all designed to help you enter the state known as BDK. The rules are simple:

♦ Eliminate all cooked food. Most importantly all cooked carbohydrates including sweets, chocolate, crisps, cake, pastas, breads, rice, potatoes, crackers and fizzy drinks. When you limit these foods you limit insulin production.

♦ In their place eat an abundance of raw plant fats – avocados, olives, young coconuts, stone pressed olive oil, nuts and seeds etc.

♦ Eat an abundance of green leafy vegetables to combine with the raw plant fats to boost your amino acid intake.

♦ Use E3Live and wheatgrass juice to heal any enzyme deficiencies.

♦ Eat soy products for the ultimate glucagon stimulating, insulin dampening effect.

♦ Lastly if you decide to eat meat (like some authorities promote), eat fresh sources of fish, foul, eggs and finally red meat.

♦ Avoid all hybrid foods that are high on the glycemic index, such as carrots, potatoes and parsnips.

♦ Minimise fruits at the start of your fat loss regime and concentrate on raw greens and raw plant fats, vegetables and sprouts. Fruit may prevent you from achieving ketosis/lipolysis in so far as they are high in carbohydrate content.

Even though the 'Kick Start Principle' helps you lose maximum amounts of weight in minimum time by restricting carbohydrate, always remember it's only a principle, not a rule carved in stone! Everything you learned from section 1 still applies, but as usual there is a time and a place for experimentation, depending on your goals. From my point of view a raw diet, whatever your choice of food will eventually strip your body of toxicity and leave you slim and vital. This principle just fine-tunes the process!

ARE YOU READY FOR THE CHALLENGE?

Regulate your insulin levels and you might as well begin the celebrations! Many people unconsciously make the association: Eating more = Getting fatter... so therefore... Eating Nothing = Maximum weight loss. WRONG! If you've ever starved yourself in an effort to lose weight, realise that all you've done is blunt your own insulin response! Yes, you probably did appear to lose weight, but at the expense of starving your body of every vital nutrient needed to survive. Not eating may appear successful to begin with because a drop in blood/insulin levels usually precedes fat loss, but once you start eating again, unchanged habits (the cause of the problem) resurface causing the classic 'yo-yo dieting' syndrome. BDK reverses this trend. Simply focus on raw plant fats, greens and soy and you'll blunt the insulin response and lose maximum amounts of fat:

- If you are incredibly obese or simply just a few stones overweight, it is likely that insulin is constantly occupying your bloodstream morning, noon and night. Excess insulin is the reason why you have put weight on and kept it on. Eliminate the cause – cooked carbohydrates.
- Sleep is a time when fatty acids and ketones are *usually* converted into fuel, but this can't take place in the presence of excess insulin!
- Insulin is a storage and locking hormone. When you kick-start your fat burning metabolism you'll stimulate glucagon and be in the fat-dissolving state.
- This fat-dissolving state known as BDK or ketosis/lipolysis is the opposite pathway to gaining fat.
- Fat Mobilisation Substance (FMS) and other lipid mobilisers are critical for kick-starting your journey. They enable you to effortlessly pass out unused calories from your body that may have been stored on your

body on the low fat, high carbohydrate diet.

♦ Feeding cooked potatoes to hogs produces rapid weight gain to ensure a higher market price.

♦ When the entry rates of carbohydrates were studied, scientists were surprised with their findings. It was thought that simple sugars enter the bloodstream quickly, whilst complex carbohydrates slowly, but studies completely disproved this. It was found that fructose (fruit sugar) enters the bloodstream more slowly than supposedly 'complex' carbohydrates such as pasta.

♦ Two other studies from the same research group in Italy indicate that excessive pasta consumption is linked to increases in colon cancer and stomach cancer. On the other hand, every major study has indicated that people who increase their consumption of fruits and vegetables reduce their risk of cancer and heart disease dramatically.

♦ There are two types of fibre, soluble and insoluble fibre. Soluble fibre includes such things as pectin, which is found in apples. Insoluble fibre includes such things as cellulose and bran found in breakfast cereals. Soluble fibre slows the entry rate of carbohydrates into your blood stream but insoluble fibre has virtually no effect.

♦ Early research conducted at the University of Toronto found that table sugar enters the bloodstream more slowly than the highly recommended breakfast cereals, such as corn flakes. You may have once thought breakfast cereal was healthy but for all intensive purposes it is nothing but pure glucose linked by chemical bonds. Once these bonds are easily broken in your stomach the glucose rushes into your bloodstream at a faster rate than the carbohydrate from table sugar. Think about the effect a daily dose of cereal has on your system.

♦ If you want to get maximum control over your insulin levels use soy. It has the advantage of causing less insulin secretion than animal protein, whilst stimulating more glucagon. A truly advantageous one-two punch in your favour! Spread your intake of protein evenly through the day.

♦ If you look into the scientific world of metabolism, you'll find the phenomenon of ketone formation documented as your major alternative fuel system. Dr George Cahill, a professor from Harvard who has respect for being a leader in the research of metabolic pathways explains how brain tissue utilises ketones more easily than glucose, being 'preferred fuel' in his opinion.

♦ Use wheatgrass juice and E3Live daily! It supplies such a cocktail of goodness you'll be on the fast track to unassailable health!

- High insulin/body fat levels increase the quantity of an enzyme that converts testosterone to oestradiol, compromising your sex drive.
- Studies have confirmed that low levels of testosterone in males correlate with an increased risk of heart disease. By lowering your insulin levels and losing body fat you indirectly decrease the quantity of the enzyme responsible for converting testosterone to oestradiol, thus maintaining optimal testosterone levels. The message: Higher insulin – lower testosterone – less sex drive! I'll let you decide how important this is!
- Twenty vegetarians can live off the land of one meat-eater.

A Final Thought: Obesity is a growing national epidemic and by losing extra fat content, you immediately jump out of a group of people who are in danger of diabetes, heart disease, stroke etc. whilst immediately jumping into an elite group of people who are living the principles of RAW PERFECTION. Come and join us!

THE RAW PERFECTION EVALUATION:
Do you want to maximise unwanted fat loss?
Have you mastered the principles of hormonal control?
Do you appreciate the role of insulin in weight gain?

If you want to know why food is more powerful than any prescription drug and how to harness this power to control every aspect of your health, pay attention. What you are about to read will fine-tune your eating habits and change the eating habits of the world.

CHAPTER 8

EICOSANOIDS:
THE POWER OF THE SUPER HORMONES

You are about to move swiftly into a different realm. A realm where cutting edge science takes over, a realm where fine-tuning is the key, and a realm that puts you in complete control of your health.

You may find this chapter very technical to begin with, so don't get too absorbed in the science of what you're about to read, simply learn what it takes to control eicosanoids (pronounced eye-car-sarnoids) and watch in awe as your entire being transforms in front of your very eyes.

All you need to know is what eicosanoids are, how they are produced, why they are critical to RAW PERFECTION, and what you can do to influence their production.

The information that follows represents the latest findings in human physiology. But hold on a minute! If what you're about to read is so ground-breaking, why haven't you heard about these super-hormones before. In fact...

IF SOME DOCTORS DON'T KNOW ABOUT EICOSANOIDS WHY SHOULD YOU?

If you've never heard of eicosanoids, don't be too concerned. Most physicians or exercise physiologists have never heard of them either. This ignorance is in spite of the fact that the 1982 Nobel Prize in Medicine was awarded to a couple of research scientists for understanding their importance in human physiology. Eicosanoids represent some of the most powerful and crucial substances in the body. They control the cardiovascular system, the immune system, and the systems that determine how much fat you store. In fact they control virtually all of your bodily functions. Yet as powerful as they are, eicosanoids are totally controlled by diet, exercise and stress.

If you asked a doctor to explain the role of eicosanoids in your body, what do you think they'd say? Do you think they'd be able to tell you that almost every prescription drug directly effects eicosanoid production in your body? Do you think they'd be able to explain why a dynamic balance of eicosanoids virtually guarantees health? Do you think they'd be able to tell you that the reason aspirin is so powerful and effective is because of its eicosanoid modulating capabilities? The reality is simple – most doctors have never heard of eicosanoids. They represent the most powerful force present within your body, and the good news is that this force is controllable. Now is your chance to...

UNCOVER THE MYSTERIES OF THE EICOSANOIDS

Why is there so much ignorance concerning the importance of eicosanoids? The answer is their complexity:

1. There are currently more than 100 known eicosanoids and more are being discovered all the time.
2. Their lifetime in the body is measured in seconds.
3. They function as 'cell to cell regulators' that rarely appear in the bloodstream.
4. They work at vanishingly low concentrations.

These facts have limited the understanding of eicosanoid biochemistry to the highest levels of medical research. This data simply has not yet filtered down to exercise physiologists, physicians or athletes.

ESSENTIAL FATTY ACIDS –
THE BUILDING BLOCKS OF POWER

Eicosanoids are derived from a unique group of polyunsaturated essential fatty acids containing 20 carbon atoms (Greek *eikosi*, twenty). Think of eicosanoids as a team of at least 100 powerful hormone-like substances responsible for the control of virtually every physiological response in your body. Like most hormones, balance is the key, but unlike most hormones eicosanoids are produced inside the cells, act inside the cells, and vanish in a fraction of a second, making them more difficult to study than endocrine hormones such as insulin and glucagon.

Once an eicosanoid is excreted by a cell, its primary objective is to test the immediate environment outside the boundaries of the cell and then report back to the cell. This information is critical and allows the cell to take appropriate biological action in response to any external alterations. By continually being sent out to assess the immediate surroundings around a cell, an eicosanoid can interact with the cell receptor on the cell surface, modifying the biological response of the cell. This complex activity has only recently been discovered, but...

EICOSANOIDS HAVE BEEN AROUND FOREVER!

Even though eicosanoids have been around for more than 500 million years, the first ones were only discovered in 1936 having been isolated from the prostate gland and named prostaglandins.

At this early stage, eicosanoids were considered another endocrine hormone using the bloodsteam to get to its target cell, but this wasn't the case, leaving scientists unable to pinpoint their role in the body. It took 40 years for any breakthrough to be made, but in the 1970s with the development of exceptionally sophisticated instrumentation, scientists were able to identify more than 100 different eicosanoids and began to identify their roles.

THE MASTER CONTROL SYSTEM

By controlling leukotrienes (another subclass of eicosanoids) you can control, among other things, bronchial constriction and allergies. By controlling and balancing prostacyclins and thromboxanes, you can control heart disease. If you modify your nutritional habits and control the production of lipoxins and hydroxylated fatty acids you'll be able to control inflammation and also regulate the immune system.

So there you have it, as each year passes, more and more eicosanoids are uncovered and categorised accordingly. Prostaglandins are the most familiar eicosanoids, but represent only a small group of this very large and powerful family. If you look at the list below you'll see what I mean. Epi-isoprostanoids were only discovered a few years before the new millennium. When controlled, they have powerful anti-cancer effects similar to those found in aspirin. Here's the list.

♦ Prostaglandins
♦ Thromboxanes
♦ Leukotrienes
♦ Lipoxins
♦ Hydroxylated fatty acids
♦ Isoprostanoids
♦ Epi-isoprostanoids
♦ Isoleukotrienes

WHY ARE YOU LEARNING ALL OF THIS?

If you can control eicosanoids, you can control the finest regulators of cellular function in existence. Imagine being able to have complete biological control over the regulation of many diverse functions, such as:

♦ blood pressure.
♦ blood clotting.
♦ the inflammation response.
♦ the immune system.
♦ uterine contractions during birth.
♦ sexual potency in men.
♦ the pain and fever response.
♦ the sleep/wake cycle.
♦ the release of gastric acid (potent new anti-ulcer drugs currently being investigated are eicosanoid modulators).
♦ the constriction and dilation of airways in the lungs and blood vessels in the tissues, and many others.

YOU'RE RESPONSIBLE FOR
THE GREATEST BALANCING ACT OF ALL

Eicosanoids are the most powerful hormones in existence and must be dynamically balanced to ensure optimal health and longevity. Imbalances of any kind, left untreated, can cause major physiological problems. This chapter will allow you to fine-tune what you've already discovered and modify your nutritional habits even more to gain control and direct the balance of these super-hormones. Take a look for yourself at the powerful roles of eicosanoids and prepare to take the reigns.

| EICOSANOID END PRODUCTS FALL INTO TWO BASIC GROUPS ||
GOOD EICOSANOIDS	BAD EICOSANOIDS
Inhibit platelet aggregation	Promote platelet aggregation
Act as vasodilators	Act as vasoconstrictors
Decrease cellular proliferation	Increase cellular proliferation
Stimulate immune response	Depress immune response
Decrease inflammation	Increase inflammation
Decrease pain transmission	Increase pain transmission
Dilate airways	Constrict airways
Increase endurance	Decrease endurance
Increase oxygen flow	Decrease oxygen flow

EICOSANOIDS – THE ACCELERATOR AND BRAKE OF OPTIMAL HEALTH

Good and bad eicosanoids are like the brake and accelerator pedals in a car. In order to pass your driving test you must master the control of both. If you put your pedal to the metal and accelerate too hard, and produce an excess of good eicosanoids, you may travel down the road to exhilarating health faster, but without the brake (bad eicosanoids) you'll lose control of the car! The bad eicosanoids can be held responsible for almost every major illness that has existed within society to date, but nevertheless, like the brake pedal in a car 'bad eicosanoids' are still necessary to get you where you want to go, even though it appears they hold you back. The reason they are labelled 'bad' is because in today's society, it's easy to engage in habits that cause their runaway production and as you know it's no good trying to drive down the road to scintillating health with your foot on the brake!

Your ultimate goal is to create a dynamic balance between 'good' and 'bad' eicosanoids and when you do, your journey towards exceptional health will be fast but steady. In fact, don't be surprised to find any unwanted rashes clearing up, allergies disappearing, joints regaining mobility, headaches vanishing, nails strengthening and asthma clearing up – This is RAW PERFECTION.

THE BENEFITS OF MAINTAINING A DYNAMIC BALANCE

Let's take a look at platelet aggregation. Platelet aggregation is the term used when platelets join together to form clumps. Good eicosanoids inhibit platelets from clumping (aggregating) and bad eicosanoids promote excessive clumping. If this clumping happens at the wrong time, a person can develop a blood clot that may lead to a heart attack or stroke. But what about if you cut yourself? If platelets lose their ability to clump together, you could bleed to death from a paper cut! Another example is blood pressure. Over production of bad eicosanoids can cause high blood pressure by constricting the arteries (i.e. vasoconstriction), but the overproduction of good eicosanoids can cause low blood pressure (i.e. vasodilation), which can lead to shock. Very few people consistently produce too many good eicosanoids! The common diseases of civilisation are the result of the production of too many bad ones. In fact, as I've said before, the bad ones aren't 'bad', but are easy to produce in a society with so many poor eating habits.

Take a look at the relationship between various illnesses and eicosanoids:

♦ Heart attack victims are making more 'bad' eicosanoids (that promote platelet aggregation and vasoconstriction) and not enough 'good' ones (that prevent platelet aggregation and promote vasodilation)

♦ High blood pressure victims are making more 'bad' eicosanoids (vasoconstrictors) and not enough 'good' ones (vasodilators).

♦ Arthritis sufferers are making more bad eicosanoids (pro-inflammatory) and fewer 'good' ones (anti-inflammatory)

♦ Cancer victims are making more 'bad' eicosanoids (immune depressing) and too few 'good' ones (immune stimulating).

♦ Sufferers of Type 2 diabetes, are making more 'bad' eicosanoids (that stimulate insulin secretion) and fewer 'good' ones (that inhibit insulin secretion).

BAD EICOSANOIDS HAVE THE POWER TO EXPOSE GENETIC PRE-DISPOSITIONS

If a group of individuals spent a lifetime producing too many bad eicosanoids, do you think they'd all show the same symptoms? Definitely not! Some may have heart disease, others cancer, whilst others may be crippled by arthritis or have diabetes. Many of these chronic diseases have a strong genetic linkage. The potential for their expression lies buried in your genes, and bad eicosanoids can expose these threats if over produced! The message is clear: In a world where 21st century breakthrough principles of health need to spread like wild fire to ensure people get control of their health again, disease can be looked upon as nothing but the body making more bad eicosanoids than good. The quality of your health is the quality of the balance between good eicosanoids and bad. Infact, the worse diet approach is one that was promoted in the later stages of the 20th Century...

THE EVILS ASSOCIATED WITH A HIGH CARBOHYDRATE DIET

Up until recently, society has encouraged a high carbohydrate diet. I used to. Years ago when I first started teaching people about nutrition, I found myself getting more and more fatigued as I forced down another bowl of pasta. I had little physical energy and my blood pressure was so high, I should have referred myself to a physician. I was playing the eicosanoid game poorly, leading to a decline in my health. Without knowing it, I was disrespecting the super-hormones that have evolved over the last 500 million years to maintain my blood sugar levels and ensure optimal health. I've learned the hard way. You don't have to! You can change your biochemistry in an instant as long as you eat in accordance with what you are about to learn. So what have you learned so far?

> ### A Quick Re-cap:
> ♦ The 1982 Nobel Prize in Medicine was awared to two research scientists for understanding the importance of eicosanoids in human physiology.
> ♦ Eicosanoids control virtually every function of your body including the cardiovascular system and immune system.
> ♦ Almost every prescription drug directly effects eicosanoids.
> ♦ Eicosanoids are derived from polyunsaturated essential fatty acids.
> ♦ Both 'good' and 'bad' eicosanoids must be kept in balance.
> ♦ A high pasta/bread/rice carbohydrate diet will thwart eicosanoid balance.

Now is the time for you to discover the secret formula for...

BUILDING EICOSANOIDS FROM SCRATCH

With the importance of eicosanoids very clear in your mind, the question is how can you control their production. Just like any construction project, you need raw materials to begin your project. It's up to you to use these raw materials to build solid foundations. Let me take you on a journey through the production of eicosanoids. Use this knowledge for the rest of your life and you'll experience the kind of legendary health that will separate you from the masses! Your immediate priority is fat! You must ensure you get enough fat in your diet – but not just any old fat – raw plant fats that provide essential fatty acids!

WITHOUT ESSENTIAL FATTY ACIDS YOU'LL NEVER PRODUCE EICOSANOIDS

For this section, I'm not going to beat around the bush. Essential fatty acids from raw plant fats are the basic raw materials needed for the eventual production of eicosanoids. Essential fatty acids can't be manufactured in the body, so therefore have to be present in the food that you eat. If you remember one thing, remember this: no essential fatty acids – no eicosanoids.

The eight essential fatty acids fall into two categories – omega 6 and omega 3 fatty acids. The eicosanoids that come from omega 3 fatty acids are relatively neutral. The eicosanoids that come from omega 6 fatty acids form the building blocks for both good and bad eicosanoids.

Stage 1. Make sure you eat a variety of raw plant fats and you will get
enough linoleic acid to begin the production of eicosanoids.

Linoleic acid is where you begin. Basically it's an essential fatty acid, an
omega 6 fatty acid to be precise. You need to ensure you include plenty
of it in your diet, so the question is: Where do you find it? Raw plant
fats. With plenty of linoleic acid present in your diet, the next stage is
transporting it into your cells somehow. Ironically this is a job for the
so-called 'bad' low-density lipoproteins (LDLs).

LOW DENSITY LIPOPROTEINS AREN'T SO BAD AFTER ALL

Whether you are familiar with 'the old cholesterol-madness mentality'
or not, LDLs used to have a very bad reputation. If you have a high LDL
to HDL ratio you increase your chance of heart disease, but having no
LDLs is also just as life threatening. If you had no LDLs you wouldn't
be able to make any eicosanoids, which ultimately is a no-win situation.
(See chapter 9 for more information about cholesterol.)

With enough linoleic acid, and a vehicle to transport it into the
eicosanoid pipeline, the next stage is getting what's available into the
production pathway so it can be converted to another fatty acid called
gamma linolenic acid (GLA). This conversion is controlled by an
enzyme, which acts like a gatekeeper, called delta 6 desaturase. You are
about to learn how to control this enzyme, because if you don't, you'll
never master control of the eicosanoid production pipeline. Imagine
linoleic acid to be the 'goods', LDLs to be the delivery lorry and delta 6
desaturase the guard that either lets you deliver your goods and convert
them into GLA or turns you away! Let's look at it in detail.

THE ENZYME STANDING AT THE GATE:
DELTA 6 DESATURASE

If delta 6 desaturase is active, you're in luck! You'll be able to deliver
your goods without any problems. If delta 6 desaturase is not active then
you'll be turned away from the gate, the entry of linoleic acid will be
denied and eicosanoid production will suffer. Your job is to do
everything possible to ensure delta 6 desaturase is active. Here's how:

VARIABLES THAT GOVERN THE ACTIVITY OF DELTA 6 DESATURASE

SPEEDS UP DELTA 6 DESATURASE	*SLOWS DOWN* DELTA 6 DESATURASE
1.Dietary Protein	1.High carbohydrate diet
	2.Trans fatty acids
	3.Alpha linoleic acid
	4.Stress
	5.Disease
	6.Ageing
	7.Zinc deficiency

DIETARY PROTEIN

Raw greens mixed with raw plant fats will supply you with the necessary amino acids to build exceptional health. Wild greens are also excellent! Soy has the best insulin dampening and glucagon stimulating qualities, making it critical food for the purposes of eicosanoid formation. The most important step in eicosanoid production is minimising the factors that slow delta 6 desaturase down. Here we go.

HIGH CARBOHYDRATE DIET

Various studies conclusively show that high carbohydrate, low protein diets inhibit the activity of delta 6 desaturase. The problem is also compounded due to the insulin producing effect of a high carbohydrate diet. This has an effect on another enzyme called delta 5 desaturase. More about that later. Alcohol is worth a mention here because its use is so widespread. It is high in sugar and interferes with the delta 6-desaturase enzyme. High sugar diets also prevent fat from being released from your own personal fat stores in your body, essentially keeping you fat! Sugar also interferes with the work of the essential fatty acids.

TRANS FATTY ACIDS

Foods that contain trans-fatty acids, especially fried foods, are dangerous to your health. They slow down the activity of delta 6 desaturase and thus inhibit the formation of good eicosanoids. Firstly they change the permeability of cell membranes, allowing unwelcome molecules in, and letting some molecules escape which would usually remain in the cell. This protective barrier is vital in keeping your cells alive and healthy. Eliminate all cooked fat and replace it with raw plant fats immediately!

Trans-fatty acids make up 37% of partially hydrogenated vegetable oils and if ingested can rapidly increase blood cholesterol level by 15% and triglyceride levels by 47%. In experiments, trans-fatty acids have been shown to have the power to increase the size of atherosclerotic plaques in the aortas of pigs. Hydrogenated oils are used in baked goods, confections such as ice cream, chocolate and sweets, and snacks such as crisps where the hydrogenated oil helps to give the product crispness. A crisp would have no crunch without the hydrogenated (hardened) oil. Eliminate them and replace them with raw plant fats!

When you look at the facts, death from cancer has increased from 1 in 30 in 1900, to over 1 in 4 in 2000. The increase parallels the increased consumption of hydrogenated vegetable oils and trans-fatty acids. Any fat that is cooked or altered is not welcome in the body.

MARGARINE MAYBE CHOLESTEROL-FREE BUT IT INCREASES CHOLESTEROL!

Margarine may be free of cholesterol, but it increases cholesterol levels because it is a potent source of trans-fatty acids. One study showed that women who ate four or more teaspoons of margarine per day had a 66% chance of contracting cardiovascular disease than women who ate about one teaspoon per month. Also, women who eat relatively high levels of the trans-fatty acids found in margarine and shortening have a much higher chance of contracting breast cancer, the number one cancer killer in women. When men eat this form of fat, they greatly increase their risk of prostate cancer. Good eicosanoids reduce the manufacture of cholesterol in the liver. Raw plant fats are the only answer!

THE IMPORTANCE OF UNDERSTANDING OILS

For oils to remain fresh and deliver vital nutrients and essential fats to the body, they must be pressed and packaged in the dark, in the absence of oxygen and heat. Having been through this kind of stringent process they must then be stored in opaque containers, excluding air and oxygen. This kind of packaging allows oils to retain their goodness for years. Alternatively, nature packages these oils in nuts and seeds, in a way that keeps light, air and heat out. Seeds can protect oils for several years without spoiling.

THE DANGERS OF HOT FAT

Many polyunsaturated fats undergo a trans-alteration during the high temperatures required for sautéing and frying, changing the molecular structure of their constituent fatty acids. Once these changes have occurred, your body finds no use for them because they can't be assimilated. Once a fat has been cooked at high temperatures, it becomes poisonous and carcinogenic (cancer causing).

Studies at the University of Helsinki, performed by Dr Rakel Kurkela showed how cooked fats can drastically reduce levels of health. He split his animal subjects into two groups:

♦ Group 1 was fed with raw, unheated safflower oil, rich in unsaturated fatty acids.
♦ Group 2 was fed with the same oil that had been heated in a frying pan.

Every other part of the diet was kept similar throughout the experiment and the results were so clear it's almost frightening. Group 1 thrived and increased their body weight. Group 2, however, deteriorated and eventually died.

When Kurkela analysed the heated oil and other unsaturated oil, he found they were filled with numerous poisonous compounds. Some of the substances found were powerful oxidisers, known for causing damage by altering the structure of cell membranes, cell nuclei and amino acids. Some other substances were cancer inducing. One such substance he discovered was malonaldehyde. Eliminate cooked fat!

ALPHA LINOLENIC ACID (ALA)

FATTY ACID PERCENTAGES OF COMMONLY USED OILS

OIL	SATURATED	MONOUNSATURATED	LA	ALA
Almond	9	65	26	0
Canola	6	60	24	10
Corn	13	27	57	2
Flaxseed	9	16	18	57
Hazelnut	7	76	16	0
Olive	10	82	8	0
Peanut	18	49	29	0
Safflower	8	13	79	0
Sesame (light)	13	46	41	0
Sunflower	12	19	69	0
Walnut	16	28	51	7

ALA is an omega-3 fatty acid found in the oils of various plants that slows down the activity of delta 6 desaturase. It should be quite apparent from the table, which oils to use and which ones to avoid. I recommend stone-pressed extra virgin olive oil. It is high in monounsaturated fats and has no ALA. As you can also see, the 'so-called' health food flaxseed and its oils are incredibly high in ALA so therefore should be eliminated or used sparingly. Many sufferers of arthritis consume flaxseeds and/or flaxseed oil to help their condition, and maybe a little confused at this point. The reason flaxseed works is because it inhibits all eicosanoid formation. It knocks out the bad ones which are causing the problem, but at the expense of preventing the formation of the good ones. This action is similar to that of aspirin.

STRESS

Stress is a word that means many things to many people. Regardless of what many authorities tend to believe, there are means and ways of accessing calm, relaxed, focused and alert state of minds without the presence of stress. Not only are there techniques that can be learned, but there are also machines that assist you in accessing peak performance brain states.

When you stop and think about it, why would you want to control stress? If you control it, the pre-supposition is that it still exists. You wouldn't want to control a dangerous old car with bad breaks and unreliable steering would you? Once you knew about its condition, you'd want a new one, or at least get it repaired. Learning to create peak performance states of mind at will, whether it be on your own, or using some of the latest brain enhancing/peak performance mind machines, is where you need to place your attention. When you use these devices or techniques, not only do you eliminate stress (a potential delta 6 desaturase inhibitor), but you also condition states of mind that can be used productively to increase the quality of your life. The hormonal benefits of relaxation training/mind machines will be covered later in chapters 11 and 12.

Back to the chase. Take a look at how stress can cause biochemical havoc in your body by overproducing the two menacing hormones...

CORTISOL AND ADRENALINE:
A PAIR OF MENACING DELTA 6 DESATURASE INHIBITORS

Stress elevates blood levels of the hormones adrenaline and cortisol.

♦ Adrenaline decreases the activity of delta 6 desaturase, and that in turn decreases the production of good eicosanoids.
♦ Cortisol increases insulin levels, leading to an over production of bad eicosanoids.

Are you beginning to see that you can be doing everything right nutritionally, but if you don't take time to relax and be quiet on the inside, you'll never master RAW PERFECTION?

Research from Harvard Medical School with 1623 cardiac patients strongly suggests that angry outbursts more than double the risk of a heart attack in the following two hours. Eliminating negative stress is a major factor in the quest to mastering eicosanoid production. In a study carried out at the Seattle Pacific Northwest Research Foundation, hundreds of rats were bred to be susceptible to breast cancer. They were then subjected to varying amounts of stress, whilst carefully monitored. The rate of cancer increased from between 7% and 92% depending on amount of stress the rats experienced. So once again, don't underestimate stress, especially with respect to eicosanoids. Some people eat poorly all their life, but manage to stay relaxed and calm, and in good spirits and live a long fun-filled life. Keep this in mind!

STRESS HORMONES AND
HORMONAL COMMUNICATION BREAKDOWN

Cortisol is the most abundant corticosteroid synthesised by your body. In excessive amounts it can accelerate ageing and cause widespread damage. The neurons in your brain are incredibly sensitive to cortisol and if exposed to increasing levels within the bloodstream, can die! If this happens continuously, the powerful feedback mechanism that controls the release of cortisol gradually breaks down and increasing amounts of cortisol are released from the adrenal glands exasperating the problem. When someone continues to damage the cortisol-sensitive neurons in their brain, cortisol secretion gradually overwhelms the body. The result: Inhibited eicosanoid formation.

Ask anyone who has taken synthetic corticosteroids for more than 30 days. After this amount of time their body goes haywire and deteriorates rapidly because they prevent any formation of eicosanoids, good or bad! Synthetic corticosteroids may appear to be doing some good initially because they knock out the production of 'bad' eicosanoids (the cause of the problem), but eventually they cause death!

DISEASE

Disease is usually a sign that your body has been under-functioning for some time. If you haven't been taking good care of yourself, you might have been creating an environment in your body that allows a virus to run you down. Viruses inhibit the action of the delta-6-desaturase enzyme, and the only known anti-viral agents are the favourable eicosanoids! The eicosanoid PGE1, is an incredibly powerful protector against viral infections, highlighting why prevention is better than cure. Viruses cause a roadblock in the eicosanoid pipeline inhibiting the activity of the delta 6-desaturase enzyme, and ultimately the production of PGE1 and other 'good' eicosanoids. You are less likely to suffer a viral infection if you engage in habits that optimise the balance of favourable eicosanoids to unfavourable eicosanoids.

AGEING

As people age, the activity of delta 6 desaturase begins to slow down, especially after 30, leaving it up to you to take responsibility to keep it active.

Age doesn't just relate to the number of years that you've been alive, it also relates to a number of other factors. There are in fact three distinct and separate ways to measure your age:

1. Chronological age – How old you are by the calendar.
2. Biological age – How old your body is in terms of critical life signs and cellular processes.
3. Psychological age – How old you feel.

Imagine being in a group of people all of similar chronological age. What would you see? Would they all look similar? Would they all act the same and have the same outlook on life? Of course not, It doesn't take a genius to realise that some people are ageing faster than normal.

HOW DO YOU SLOW DOWN THE AGEING PROCESS?

It is safe to say that you can't change your chronological age, but you can change your biological age. All you need to do is take a look at the list of biological parameters that determine how fast various systems of your body are ageing, and then reverse these parameters. Through the process of ageing the following biological markers alter to some degree. Take a look for yourself:

◆ Insulin resistance increases.
◆ Systolic blood pressure increases.
◆ Body fat percentage and lipid ratios increase.
◆ Glucose tolerance decreases.
◆ Aerobic capacity decreases.
◆ Muscle mass and strength decreases.
◆ Temperature regulation decreases in efficiency.
◆ Immune function diminishes.

It's worth pointing out that this fairly broad list of physiological changes can all be related to one single factor – excess insulin production. Need I say more! By combining the very best nutritional principles present within these pages, backed up with aerobic exercise, anaerobic exercise and the use of the latest developments in mind technology, you'll live a long youthful life, maintaining an optimal eicosanoid balance.

Psychological age is also a very powerful factor, which is influenced by many interweaving personal and social factors. Here is a list of questions you may like to ask yourself. Regardless of your answers, it would be worth asking yourself how you could improve each one and therefore increase the level of your psychological health.

How happy are you in your marriage or existing relationship?
How happy are you within your present job?
How happy are you within yourself?
How satisfying is your sex life?
How good is your ability to make and keep close friends?
How regular is your daily routine?
How regular is your work routine?
Do you take at least one week's vacation per year?
How much control do you feel you have over your personal life?
How much do you enjoy leisure time and your hobbies?
How easy do you find it to express your feelings?
How optimistic are you about the future?
How financially secure are you?
How much do you enjoy living within your means?

When you read chapter 17 – The Parameters of Success, you'll read an amazing story of how a group of people reversed every biological marker of ageing simply by changing their environment and their perception of reality! But for now let's get back to the eicosanoid production pipeline.

ZINC DEFICIENCY

Zinc deficiency, which is widespread, slows down the delta 6-desaturase enzyme. Every vital nutrient must be included in your diet to prevent viral infections, weak tissues and a weak immune system. The importance of having a base-line standard where you consume nutrient rich raw foods, minimising cellular stress and maximising waste elimination, can never be under-estimated. If you have white spots on your nails it's likely you have zinc deficiency. The best way to increase your zinc uptake is to include E3Live in your diet. Dr Gillian McKeith, in her book 'Miracle Superfood: Wild Blue-Green Algae' tells the remarkable story of how zinc capsules, tablets, lozenges or zinc liquid did nothing to improve her condition of zinc deficiency. The only food that eliminated the white spots and restored her zinc levels to normal was AFA blue-green algae. I suggest you buy the book and begin to use E3Live daily.

LET THE STRUGGLE COME TO A GRINDING HALT

You've covered just about everything that inhibits Delta 6 desaturase. You should now have a fair idea why many people struggle with their health. They live in stress, eat a high carbohydrate diet, use margarine and other foods with high levels of trans-fatty acids and cook oil causing it to become carcinogenic.

By applying the principle of RAW PERFECTION, you'll eat green leafy vegetables, raw plant fats, fibrous fruits and vegetables and include wheatgrass juice and/or E3Live daily. It's hard to feel stress when your body is operating so perfectly!

Take a look at the table again and get a sense of what you've just discovered. It's easy to see why many people engage in habits that result in the inactivity of the enzyme delta 6 desaturase.

VARIABLES THAT GOVERN THE ACTIVITY OF DELTA 6 DESATURASE

SPEEDS UP DELTA 6 DESATURASE	*SLOWS DOWN* DELTA 6 DESATURASE
1.Dietary Protein	1.High carbohydrate diet
	2.Trans fatty acids
	3.Alpha linoleic acid
	4.Stress
	5.Disease
	6.Ageing
	7.Zinc deficiency

At this point I suggest you take a break. You've learned a great deal already and it's worth re-reading the first part of this chapter or at least skimming over it to refresh your memory. Essentially, linoleic acid is supplied via raw plant fats and transported via LDL cholesterol into the eicosanoid production pathway. Linoleic acid needs to be converted into gamma linoleic acid (GLA) and the activity of the enzyme delta-6 desaturase determines how fast this conversion takes place. The activity is controlled by the factors in the previous table. The next stages of eicosanoid production are critical, so when you come back from your well-earned break, prepare for...

THE VITAL CONVERSION:
LINOLEIC ACID – TO – GAMMA LINOLEIC ACID (GLA)

So far we've done everything to maximise the activity of delta 6 desaturase. We've taken the abundant amounts of Linoleic acid and followed some simple guidelines to keep the gatekeeper 'delta 6 desaturase' active. Linoleic acid has now burst into the eicosanoid production pathway and is ready for action!

At this point delta 6 desaturase converts the linoleic acid into a more metabolically activated fatty acid known as gamma linoleic acid (GLA). What is so special about GLA? GLA is the result of the body's first biochemical step, transforming the essential fatty acids into eicosanoids. GLA is an activated essential fatty acid, and tiny amounts enter the metabolic pipelines allowing the body to make other activated essential fatty acids. Your body's metabolic pipeline must be filled with enough GLA to allow eicosanoid production to be efficient.

AFA ALGAE AND THE GLA CONNECTION

If delta 6 desaturase is inhibited, you can supply GLA directly to your cells by including E3Live in your diet. AFA algae is rich in GLA. This is one of the reasons it helps to combat many conditions of poor health. Usually when eicosanoid production is compromised, illness and disease are given the chance to run rampant, but with the inclusion of GLA, the eicosanoid production pathway can continue to some degree.

SUCKLING ON THE BOSOM OF HEALTH:
THE MOTHER'S MILK CONNECTION

Since delta 6 desaturase doesn't reach full activity until six months after birth, how does a baby ensure adequate levels of GLA are present in their eicosanoid production pipeline? Answer: By drinking mother's milk! Whether you've just given birth or are planning a pregnancy, the quality of the milk you supply your offspring makes a tremendous difference to the quality of their health. But the quality of your milk is only as good as the quality of the nutrition you feed yourself. Make sure you supply enough nutrition for yourself and your baby, regardless of whether you decide to breast feed or not. Remember a healthy baby is a happy baby! Note: If you are pregnant, wait until your baby is born before you begin the use of E3Live. If you don't take this advice, ensure you only use ¼ teaspoon daily.

So where are you now in your level of understanding?

♦ LDL cholesterol transports linoleic acid into cells.
♦ The gatekeeper enzyme, delta 6 desaturase allows linoleic acid to be converted to gamma linolenic acid (GLA) and AFA algae contains GLA helping the equation.
♦ The next stage in the pipeline is for GLA to be converted to another fatty acid dihomo gamma linolenic acid (DGLA). This is a rapid process if you have enough GLA in your system to begin with, so we'll move swiftly on!

Now you are at a critical cross-roads. Your decision about what to eat will determine whether you make 'good' eicosanoids or 'bad' eicosanoids.

STANDING AT THE CROSSROADS
WITH DELTA 5 DESATURASE

Having followed the process meticulously up until now, there are two potential routes that DGLA can take. One path will lead to the production of 'good' eicosanoids and the other path will lead to the production of 'bad' eicosanoids. The key factor that determines which metabolic pathway will be chosen is controlled by another enzyme. The enzyme is called delta 5 desaturase.

♦ If delta 5 desaturase is activated, DGLA will be converted into another activated essential fatty acid: arachidonic acid (AA), and then towards 'bad' eicosanoid formation.
♦ If delta 5 desaturase is inhibited, your body will produce more DGLA and form 'good' eicosanoids.

In the early stages you wanted to increase the activity of delta 6 desaturase. Now you want to minimise the activity of delta 5 desaturase. Confused? You ought to be!

Now, if you can inhibit delta 5 desaturase and promote the production of 'good' eicosanoids you can...

PREPARE FOR THE UNLIMITED
HEALTH BENEFITS OF PGE1

The series 1 prostaglandins made from DGLA are the most famous eicosanoids. Although they've all been studied in depth, the most famous one is prostaglandin E1, or PGE1. PGE1 has a myriad of important functions in your body. To begin with, it keeps blood platelets from sticking together, helping to prevent heart attacks and strokes caused by blood clots in the arteries. It assists the kidneys by helping to remove fluid from the body, acting as a diuretic. It opens up blood vessels, improves circulation and helps to relieve angina. It slows down cholesterol production. It prevents inflammation and controls arthritis. It makes insulin work more effectively, helping diabetics. It improves nerve function and will give you a consistent emotional high. It regulates calcium metabolism. It is involved in the functioning of the T-cells of the immune system, which destroy foreign cell invasions. It may also help to prevent cancer cell growth by regulating the rate of cell division. Finally PGE1 prevents the release of arachidonic acid (AA) from cell membranes. This is important for reasons you are about to discover.

THE CRITICAL INSULIN AND GLUCAGON LINK:
INHIBITING DELTA 5 DESATURASE

If you want to ensure you get all the benefits from PGE1 and the other favourable eicosanoids, your goal: Inhibit delta 5 desaturase. How? Disengage any habits that allow the over production of insulin and include E3Live in your nutritional regime as it contains the essential fatty EPA (eicosapentaenoic acid). EPA directly inhibits the activity of delta 5 desaturase. Let's re-cap:

♦ Insulin activates delta 5 desaturase. It's up to you to control its production!

♦ Glucagon inhibits delta 5 desaturase. Ensure you eat quality protein sources to stimulate glucagon!
♦ The omega-3 essential fatty acid EPA also inhibits delta 5 desaturase. It can be found in E3Live.

Need I say more! The positive balance of DGLA to AA sets up whether or not 'good' or 'bad' eicosanoids predominate. By following the principles of RAW PERFECTION you'll be maximising the dynamic balance of eicosanoids and ensuring a vital life.

WHERE THE FORK IN THE CROSS-ROADS TAKES YOU AND WHY ARACHIDONIC ACID IS YOUR BIOLOGICAL NIGHTMARE

You were at the crossroads. One path took you towards more DGLA and good eicosanoids, such as PGE1. The other path took you towards arachidonic acid and bad eicosanoids. Let's discover more about the effects of arachidonic acid (AA) and how this essential fatty acid can be your worst enemy. Just as AA is essential to life, it is also destructive in excessive amounts. It is so dangerous that when injected into laboratory animals, they die within minutes. Other fatty acids can be injected into the same laboratory animals with no ill effects. AA is the precursor of bad eicosanoids.

WHERE CAN YOU FIND ARACHIDONIC ACID?

AA is found in all meats, especially red meats and organ meats and in egg yolks. These foods get a hard time for their saturated fat and cholesterol content. But most of the problems actually stem from the AA content – especially to those individuals who are sensitive to it.

Too much AA (or a distinct sensitivity to it) causes a variety of symptoms such as chronic fatigue, poor sleep, grogginess upon awakening, brittle hair and nails, constipation, minor rashes and dry, flaking skin. If these are symptoms that you've been experiencing at any point, then continue mastering the principles of RAW PERFECTION. Greens, raw plant fats, fruits and vegetables are the only answer!

EVALUATE YOUR HEALTH
EVALUATE YOUR EICOSANOID STATUS

♦ **Energy and Performance** – As levels of DGLA increase and more 'good' eicosanoids are produced, you increase oxygen transfer and begin to make better use of stored body fat, leading to more energy and increased performance. An increase in tiredness can be associated with the production of too many 'bad' eicosanoids or too much AA in the diet.

♦ **Refined Carbohydrate Cravings** – As you begin to use raw greens, raw plant fats, fruits and vegetables to your advantage in meals, juices, smoothies or on their own, you'll limit the production of bad eicosanoids, and establish optimal eicosanoid balance. Carbohydrate cravings will vanish!

♦ **Length of time of appetite suppression** – Inhibiting insulin secretion is critical when it comes to controlling hunger, so use raw plant fats to slow the release of sugar into your bloodstream. This will also keep eicosanoid formation balanced and neuropeptide Y synthesis low enough for you to suppress your appetite naturally. By supplying so many high quality nutrients you won't even feel hungry.

♦ **Finger nail and hair strength** – As you increase the production of 'good' eicosanoids, such as PGE1, you automatically increase the structural protein keratin. Keratin is the principle structural component of fingernails and hair. If you've suffered from brittle fingernails in the past, or weak hair, it is likely that you've been creating too many 'bad' eicosanoids, decreasing keratin synthesis.

♦ **Sleeping patterns** – One of the main reasons you need sleep is to re-establish neurotransmitter equilibrium. You can speed this process up by producing more 'good' eicosanoids, lessening your need for sleep. This is the main reason you don't want to eat a big meal before bedtime. The excess insulin can cause an increase in 'bad' eicosanoid formation, increasing sleep needs and making you feel groggy when you wake up.

♦ **Feeling of well being** – As you maintain optimal eicosanoid balance, you are likely to feel excellent on a more consistent basis. The over production of 'bad' eicosanoids generally leads to depression, anxiety and irritability.

♦ **Brain state** – Keeping your blood sugar levels constant will maximise your chances of maintaining exceptional concentration.

♦ **Skin beauty** – As you increase the production of 'good' eicosanoids and maintain the optimal balance, you'll begin to develop beautiful skin. Eczema and skin dryness is caused by too many bad eicosanoids (leukotrienes). 'Good' eicosanoids promote collagen synthesis, increase microcirculation and are anti-inflammatory.

THE MASTER FORMULA FOR RAW PERFECTION

If you want to learn more about the importance of eicosanoid control, read 'The Zone' books by Dr Barry Sears. These are some of the finest nutritional books on the market, and will reinforce the principles of nutrition for hormonal control. Many people instinctively know that their diet should be balanced. When people say "I fancy this for dinner tonight, or I fancy that" they are sometimes making choices based on their subconscious needs to re-establish balance of some kind. Unfortunately, most people choose recreational foods instead of powerful raw alternatives, further exasperating imbalances on a biochemical level. The Zone Diet is a best-selling approach that addresses the issue of balance very specifically. Dr. Barry Sears' Zone Diet balances carbohydrates, fats and proteins in a 40:30:30 ratio respectively, optimising eicosanoid production. Suprisingly, he doesn't make the distinction between cooked food and raw organic plant foods. He does say in one of his latest books that 'The Soy Zone' is the healthiest 'Zone' yet! In 'The Soy Zone' Soy products replace meat and dairy products as the glucagon stimulating source of protein. It wouldn't surprise me if Barry Sears writes a final book called, 'The Raw Zone'! If you want to optimise eicosanoid balance on a diet of raw foods alone, your primary mentality will be to utilise the power of green leafy vegetables, raw plant fats and organic fruits/sprouts and vegetables.

BALANCING THE TERRIFIC TRIO
HOW TO LIVE BY THE RAW PERFECTION PRINCIPLES

Your basic formula for optimal eicosanoid formation and scintillating health is to balance:
1.Chlorophyll-rich green leafy vegetables (wild greens being the best)
2.High water content sugar fruits (melons, tropical/subtropical fruits, etc.)
3.Fats (avocados, coconuts, nuts, seeds, olives, durians, etc)

Any imbalance in the body will have its roots in a deficiency of one or more of the above foods. Anyone failing on a raw food diet must immediately ask themselves whether or not they are balancing greens, sugars and raw plant fats. Remember, cooked food is dead. Raw plant food is all-powerful. If you can balance your consumption of green leafy vegetables, fruits and fats, you'll immediately begin to appreciate the power they have over your body and before long you'll have complete dominance over your diet and health.

MAKING THE THREE MASTER FOODS WORK FOR YOU
YOUR MISSION: CREATE ULTIMATE RAW FOOD BALANCE

Once you can recognise chlorophyll-rich green foods, such as spinach, kale, parsely etc, and raw plant fats, such as nuts, seeds, durians, olives, avocados etc. and fruits/sprouts etc., you can systematically revolutionise your approach to food.

To get you started, here's a brief look at how you'll begin thinking and acting:

♦ An abundance of green leafed vegetables must be backed up with sweet fruits and raw plant fats. The more stimulating the green leafed vegetables, (i.e. kale) the stronger the sweet fruits and fatty foods must be to maintain balance. The less stimulating the green-leafed vegetables (i.e. romaine lettuce), the less stimulating the sweet fruits and fatty foods need to be. Simple.

♦ A strong fat (avocado) is best balanced by deeper green-leaves. One of my favourite drinks is to juice half a head of celery with 2-3 apples and 350g of kale, then pour the juice in a blender with 150g of spinach, an avocado and a chilli pepper. It's thick, it's heavy and it fills me up for hours!

♦ A strong sugar (banana) balances well with heavier fats (nuts), which themselves also balance well with dark green-leafed vegetables in the same day. Another favourite of mine is to mash up a banana and mix it with a handful of blended nuts. Remember the simpler the combination and the less foods used the better. To begin with do whatever you want as long as it's raw!

BALANCE YOURSELF NATURALLY WITH
NON STIMULATING FOODS

The only foods that aren't part of the all-powerful trio are non-sweet fruits. These foods are neutral and will keep you balanced on a pinnacle of health. Cucumbers are an excellent example.

The least stimulating foods on the human body are low sugar, low fat, high water content foods, but that doesn't mean you should only eat these. Variety plays a critical part in a high raw diet.

Non-sweet fruits are low stimulation foods and include: **bell peppers (not green) breadfruit, cranberry, cucumber, courgette, dragon fruit, grapefruit, jalapeno pepper, lemon, lime, noni, okra, pumpkin, serrano pepper, summer squashes, tomatillo and tomato.**

THE GOLDEN RULE: EAT MORE ABUNDANTLY THOSE
FOODS HIGH IN WATER CONTENT

The more you eat a balance of raw greens, fats, and fruits, the more you'll realise how powerful they are. From time to time, isolate one food and allow it to dominate your diet for a few days. This will give you first hand experience of the power of raw plant food. If you are not experimenting, never leave greens, sweet fruits or raw fats out of your diet! Consider digestion as well, you may be more comfortable eating certain foods together and others apart. Perfection would be to only eat one type of food at any one sitting. For those of you who want to experiment with mono-dieting, be my guest.

If you trust my word and I hope you do, the best path to take is that of experimentation. You'll automatically develop powerful references and sharpen your intuition!

You have a simple feedback mechanism if you want to succeed. If you feel you haven't had enough greens, create a spinach/kale/apple juice drink and enjoy. If you've missed out on fats in a day, eat some olives, avocados, nuts or seeds. If you think you've overdosed on sugar concentrate on fats and greens to balance. By tuning your mind to these three food classes you'll be on the fast track to nutritional supremacy.

USING JUICING TO YOUR ADVANTAGE

Juicing is a very powerful tool in your raw food arsenal. There are many juicers on the market. When buying one, my criteria is based on how easy it is to clean! Many authorities are too interested in promoting ones that maximise nutrient extraction. This is fine if you have the time to clean it, but since I juice greens quite often, I prefer ones that are convenient! Complicated juicers may extract more nutrients, but if you can't be bothered to use it, it'll be a waste of space.

If you haven't heard of Jay Kordich, you need to buy his book immediately, entitled 'The Juiceman'. In the late 1940s, he conducted an experiment on 65 prisoners suffering from stomach ulcers. The majority of his treatment involved feeding them cabbage juice, which is saturated with the amino acid glutamine. Within only three weeks, 63 of his subjects were completely cured and the other two only had minimal symptoms. Cabbage has sometimes been called the king of the cruciferous family. It is alkalinising, cleansing, rejuvenating, contains substantial amounts of sulphur, iodine, iron, vitamins C and E. It also happens to be one of the cheapest vegetables. Always over-estimate the power of juicing!

VEGETARIANS, VEGANS, EXCESSIVE WEIGHT AND TIREDNESS

If you've been sold on the idea of being vegetarian or vegan and suffer with unwanted body fat and tiredness, begin to learn how to balance raw greens, raw fats and raw sugars, the results will astound you! Be warned, onlookers will be suspicious at your vitality and lust for life. You may slip back to old habits from time to time, but as long as you're aware of what causes you to feel fabulous on a consistent basis, you'll be sure to return.

The Bulgarians have an incredible reputation for longevity, sometimes reaching ages of up to 125 years and with a diet of fruits (sugar), vegetables (chlorophyll), and sour milk or buttermilk (fat) it's easy to see why. They've found a near perfect balance.

I want you to have a reason – why you eat – what you eat – when you eat it. With this knowledge you'll be able to anticipate and design the result you want, leading to mastery. Some people say it's too technical, but so is driving a car until you master it. People never question learning to drive because their life depends on it. I think your life depends more on your diet and health than your ability of move a metal box around a strip of tarmac. Some people say it takes the spontaneity out of eating, yet 90% of their meals are probably the same week in and week out, they just don't notice it because they don't pay attention to it.

ARE YOU READY FOR THE CHALLENGE?

As your metabolism begins to burn fat rather than carbohydrate, you'll need more water than usual on a daily basis, because good eicosanoids increase water flow to the colon. Ensure you keep your raw food intake high and you'll be in total control. If however you find that you are suffering with constipation, even after eating many high-water content raw foods, you are probably releasing stored arachidonic acid from fat cells. For about 25% of the population, there will be a transitory release of stored arachidonic acid from stored body fat. This build up will be a direct result of old dietary habits, and can give rise to constipation by reducing water flow into the colon. If you are eating an abundance of raw greens, raw plant fats, fruit and vegetables, the problems will be short-lived.

I appreciate this was not the easiest of chapters to read and will take you time to master, so here is a re-cap.

♦ Eicosanoids control all of your body functions including your cardiovascular system, immune system, and how much fat you store!
♦ Most prescription drugs have a direct effect on eicosanoid production. The reason aspirin is so powerful and effective is because of its eicosanoid modulating capabilities.
♦ Use the nutritional distinctions in this chapter and you'll have control over your blood pressure, blood clotting, the inflammation response, your immune system, uterine contractions during birth, sexual potency, the pain and fever response, the sleep/wake cycle, the release of gastric acid (potent new anti-ulcer drugs now under investigation are eicosanoid modulators), the constriction and dilation of airways in the lungs and blood vessels in the tissues, and many others.
♦ Heart attack victims are making more 'bad' eicosanoids (that promote platelet aggregation and vasoconstriction) and not enough 'good' ones (that prevent platelet aggregation and promote vasodilation).
♦ High blood pressure victims are making more 'bad' eicosanoids

(vasoconstrictors) and not enough 'good' ones (vasodilators).

♦ Arthritis sufferers are making more bad eicosanoids (pro-inflammatory) and fewer 'good' ones (anti-inflammatory).

♦ Cancer victims are making more 'bad' eicosanoids (immune depressing) and too few 'good' ones (immune stimulating).

♦ Sufferers of Type II diabetes, are making more 'bad' eicosanoids (that stimulate insulin secretion) and fewer 'good' ones (that inhibit insulin secretion).

♦ Essential fatty acids are the basic raw materials needed to produce eicosanoids. Essential fatty acids can't be manufactured in the body, so therefore have to be present in the food that you eat.

♦ Linoleic acid is your starting point. It's an omega 6 essential fatty acid and found in virtually every food. With enough in your diet the part of cholesterol known as low-density lipoproteins (LDLs) will transport it to the eicosanoid production pipeline. An enzyme known as delta 6 desaturase determines whether or not linoleic acid enters the eicosanoid production pathway, acting like a gatekeeper. Speed up its activity and you are on your way to unassailable health. Slow it down and the problems begin.

♦ Delta 6 desaturase also converts the linoleic acid into a more metabolically activated fatty acid known as gamma linolenic acid (GLA). A substance found in abundance in mothers' milk and E3Live. Babies don't produce it until they are six months old. Potential mothers take note!

♦ GLA then gets converted into another fatty acid known as Dihomo Gamma Linolenic acid (DGLA). This is a rapid process if you have enough GLA in your system.

♦ You are now at the crossroads: If delta 5 desaturase is activated, DGLA will be converted into another activated essential fatty acid: arachidonic acid (AA), and then towards bad eicosanoid formation.

♦ If delta 5 desaturase is inhibited, your body will produce more DGLA and form 'good' eicosanoids. Your goal: Inhibit this enzyme by controlling insulin and glucagon.

♦ The Omega-3 essential fatty acid EPA also inhibits delta 5 desaturase and can be found in AFA algae. Ensure you begin your life-long-love of E3Live TODAY!

♦ Do your best to limit the production of arachidonic acid and minimise its presence in your diet. It's found in all meats, especially red meats and organ meats and egg yolks. Too much AA may cause chronic fatigue, poor sleep, grogginess upon awakening, brittle hair and nails, constipation, minor rashes and dry, flaking skin.

♦ Remember the magic formula for success with RAW PERFECTION is to balance green leafy plant foods, raw plant fats and fruits, optimising eicosanoid control.

So there you have it. The distinctions in this chapter can catapult you to unprecedented success. YOUR health is in YOUR hands. Make your choices wisely and a life of freedom awaits you.

THE RAW PERFECTION EVALUATION:
Are you eating a healthy supply of raw plant fats?
Are you doing all you can to keep delta 6 desaturase active?
Are you doing all you can to keep delta 5 desaturase inactive?
Are you balancing raw plant fats, greens and fruits?

CHAPTER 9

FURTHER DOWN THE ROAD OF INSULIN EXCESS

Imagine a society free from obesity. Imagine if diabetes and blood sugar abnormalities no longer plagued millions of people. Imagine no-one suffering from elevated cholesterol levels. Imagine if high blood pressure was a problem of the past and the number 1 killer, heart disease, was eradicated for good! Do you think this is a crazy dream? It isn't when you realise that they are all symptoms of one problem: Insulin excess. Each of these so-called health disorders are nothing but messages from your body telling you to STOP ENGAGING IN HABITS THAT OVER-STIMULATE INSULIN. Each and every day, advertisers are attempting to influence you to eat more recreational foods and drink more alcohol! Moderation is one thing, addiction is another! If you don't use what you've learnt in this book to expand and extend the range of your own healthy habits, recreational foods will become the mainstay of your diet and insulin will rob you of your health. Be warned!

THE DEADLY JOURNEY FROM INSULIN RESISTANCE TO TYPE II DIABETES

If you continue to over-stimulate insulin you put yourself at risk of developing Type II diabetes. It's not something you develop overnight, it's more insidious than that. Rather than call it a disease, or even a symptom of hyperinsulinemia, think of it as a last ditch effort from your body to communicate to you that your current habits are destroying your health! It's up to you to...

HEAR THE MESSAGE AND RESPOND

A genetically susceptible person may spend their childhood consuming all kinds of insulin-inducing junk, (sweets, crisps, chocolate, fizzy drinks) and look fine on the outside! But as time goes by, the onslaught of sugar, saturated fat and toxicity is doing nothing but laying the foundation for a future of disastrous health! A child or teenager may appear to be riding 'high' on a diet of recreational foods, but with insulin occupying their bloodstream morning, noon and night, the foundation is set for future problems. As the insulin sensors in their tissues become overwhelmed by the constant influx of insulin, gradually they develop a mild form of insulin-resistance. The sensors then become less and less sensitive and the pancreas has to produce more and more insulin to keep blood sugar levels under control. If it doesn't the excess sugar can damage the brain. Normal blood sugar levels are approximately 60mg/dl to 120mg/dl (mg/dl means milligrams of glucose in 100 millilitres of blood), and very high levels, such as 800, can lead to coma and death. Insulin prevents blood sugar levels from rising too high, making it an important part of your hormonal balancing act, but as you know, this is only half the story.

OVER-TIRED AND STRESSED? ARE YOU FIGHTING THE BATTLE OF BLOOD-SUGAR ABNORMALITIES?

Have you ever wondered why overweight people are tired so much of the time? As more and more insulin is secreted in response to a poor diet, the insulin receptors on the surfaces of the cells become blocked from carrying out their function. This stops insulin from stimulating the transfer of glucose to the cells for energy use.

Although insulin lowers blood glucose levels, it can do so too efficiently causing blood sugar to fall too rapidly. This can lead to hypoglycaemia. The symptoms of hypoglycaemia can include depression, dizziness, crying spells, aggression, insomnia, lack of sexual interest and blackouts.

Not only are fat people tired because their cells are not effectively taking in energy, but throughout the day, they are the victims of hypoglycaemia, or low blood sugar, the ironic consequence of consuming *too* much sugar!

WARNING: INSULIN EXCESS CAN EXCITE THE DEADLY STRESS HORMONE

Excess insulin also inhibits the release of glucagon. Glucagon's job is to restore blood sugar levels for optimal brain function. If glucagon secretion is inhibited, your body has to release cortisol from the adrenal glands in an effort to restore blood glucose levels. If this cycle continues the adrenal glands can burn out, your ability to deal with stress weakens and your ability to raise blood sugar levels declines, resulting in hypoglycaemia again! All because of over-consumption of refined sugars! The picture isn't pretty is it!?

AN UGLY SITUATION: REACHING BURNOUT

When severe insulin resistance takes hold of its victim, the pancreas is forced to release copious amounts of insulin in an effort to regulate blood sugar levels. If the situation gets worse and the insulin sensors continue to malfunction, there comes a point when their pancreas is working at maximum capacity. This is the critical point. If nothing is done to improve the situation the insulin sensors continue to lose sensitivity and eventually the pancreas can't produce enough insulin to control blood sugar levels. Gradually the patient's blood sugar status reaches diabetic levels. At this point Type II diabetes is just around the corner. We'll get back to that shortly. For now…

A BRIEF INSIGHT INTO TYPE I DIABETES

Just to sidetrack for a moment. In type I diabetes, a virus or other toxic substance destroys the insulin-producing cells in the pancreas, and the victim requires treatment with insulin injections. It usually develops in childhood or adolescence. You can imagine what happens can't you? With no insulin being produced, glucagon causes fat to pour rapidly out of the fat cells and into the blood, putting a heavy burden on the liver. In contrast to other cells, liver mitochondria process fatty acids differently. They don't burn the fatty acids for energy, but instead partially break them down into molecules called ketone bodies, and release them into circulation. Ketone bodies are a good source of fuel for the brain and can also be burned for energy by muscle and other tissues, or eliminated via bladder, bowels or breath. Ketone bodies, however, are acids and if too many accumulate in the blood, the blood becomes more and more acidic, throwing the acid/alkaline balance into turmoil. If this continues untreated, the victim experiences the metabolic nightmare known as diabetic ketoacidosis, often leading to coma and death. With this kind of metabolic disaster it's easy to see why an undiagnosed victim can lose 30 or 40 pounds in a month or two, regardless of their increased food intake. They will often experience uncontrollable hunger.

The similarities that exist between Type I and Type II diabetes, include:

♦ Sugar spillage into the urine.
♦ Frequent urination.
♦ A great thirst.
♦ Increased blood glucose, which causes degenerative complications of the eyes, nerves, kidneys, and blood vessels.

THE LINK BETWEEN TYPE I AND TYPE II DIABETES

Back to Type II diabetes. When someone has spent a lifetime eating an abundance of insulin inducing foods (refined carbohydrates and convenience 'junk' food) their chronic blood-insulin levels eventually dampen the sensitivity of the insulin sensors. This continual cycle pushes the pancreas to its limit. It can no longer produce enough insulin to restore optimal blood/glucose levels. Glucose at high blood concentrations is toxic to the brain and many other tissues, including the pancreatic beta cells that produce the insulin. After many years, if excessive glucose has over-stimulated the insulin producing beta cells, they can fatigue/burnout and ultimately stop producing insulin altogether.

THIS IS WHERE BIOCHEMICAL TURMOIL REALLY SETS IN

As long as the beta cells can produce insulin, the deadly ketoacidosis of Type I diabetes is avoided. But if enough beta cells fatigue and insulin production falls sufficiently, glucagon takes the reigns and the balance shifts in the opposite direction causing the problems of Type I diabetes to prevail. In normal circumstances the beta cells continue to produce just enough insulin to keep ketoacidosis at bay.

Under the supervision of a physician, even those with Type I diabetes can significantly lower their insulin doses and attain much better control over their blood sugar levels by concentrating on raw, enzyme rich foods. They must also eliminate the 'junk foods' that caused the blood sugar highs and lows in the first place. Many people have completely regenerated their pancreas with the use of raw food and over time eliminated the need for insulin!

RAW PERFECTION HEALS THE PERILS OF A COOKED DIET

Raw chlorophyll has been used to treat diabetes. It acts as a catalyst allowing for greater absorption of nutrients essential for metabolising sugar. Acidic blood can be a serious problem for sufferers of diabetes and is usually the result of a diet excessive in recreational foods. Chlorophyll has a strong alkalising effect, helping to combat this condition. With a weakened pancreas, if chlorophyll is derived from E3Live or wheatgrass juice, it will also contain blood sugar balancing nutrients like chromium, magnesium and zinc. Both E3Live and wheatgrass juice encourage cell renewal for the restoration of the weakened pancreas. The three nutrients chromium, magnesium and zinc also help to restore the sensitivity of insulin receptor sites that need to remain highly sensitive in order to assist in the regulation of insulin.

ENZYME RICH RAW FOODS CONTROL INSULIN
RESTORING OPTIMAL HEALTH

The great Albert Schweitzer was a severe diabetic and when he decided to get help from the raw food pioneer Max Gerson, he was incredibly ill and injecting mega doses of insulin. The first change Gerson made to Schwietzer's diet was to eliminate cooked protein. Excessive protein relies on enzymes produced by the pancreas for its breakdown. The pancreas also secretes insulin and glucagon. In this case it needed to be rested and given the chance to regenerate, so its functions could be restored. A poor functioning pancreas is partly responsible for diabetes, and if you overtax it by eating a diet excessively high in protein you'll only make matters worse. To restore flagging enzyme levels and put even less strain on the pancreas Gerson put Schweitzer on a regime of fresh raw vegetables and lots of vegetable and fruit juices, including apple juice. Some schools of thought are against fresh fruit juices because they are high on the glycemic index (see appendix), it's worth repeating that one shouldn't judge all carbohydrates as equal, since fresh apple juice, with all its fruit sugar, quite obviously helped Schwietzer's return to health. Only ten days after this intervention, Gerson judged it safe to reduce his patient's insulin intake by half and only one month later Schwietzer needed no insulin at all. His diabetes never returned and he remained healthy and very active until his death in 1965 at the age of 92. Raw foods have the power to control insulin and rebuild a weak, almost lifeless body.

WHERE ELSE CAN HYPERINSULINEMIA CHIP AWAY AT HEALTH? INSULIN INCREASES THE PRESSURE

Hypertension is the term used for high blood pressure, and once again, excess insulin is the cause. If you've ever suffered with high blood pressure, treat it as a message that your health is in need of repair. There are three ways that hyperinsulinemia causes hypertension.

1. Hyperinsulinemia causes fluid retention

Imagine the bloodstream as a superhighway that runs throughout the body delivering nutrients to cells, whilst simultaneously assisting in the elimination of waste. What most people fail to realise is that the blood also bathes cells with electrolytes allowing the critical functions of the cell to operate as effortlessly as possible. Sodium, potassium, chloride, bicarbonate, and other substances must be maintained within a strict zone to maintain optimal cellular function. But how is this done? In step the kidneys. They act like filters and ensure that waste products are removed and the concentration of electrolytes remains balanced.

THE INCREDIBLE BALANCING ACT

If too much sodium is present at any one time in the blood, the kidneys filter it out. It gets sent to the bladder to be removed via your urine. If there isn't enough sodium, your kidneys hold onto as much of it as they can, whilst removing enough fluid to encourage optimal blood-sodium concentration.

The role of diuretics is to force the kidneys to eliminate more sodium than usual, which then causes excess fluid to be eliminated allowing blood concentrations of sodium to remain in a tight zone.

Insulin, however, forces the kidneys to retain sodium no matter what the circumstances, and since the sodium concentration must be kept in a tight zone, the kidneys retain excess fluid in order to dilute the excess sodium. The equation is simple: More insulin = more sodium retention = more fluid retention. With body fluids rising and blood volume increasing, it's easy to see how blood pressure increases, reaching dangerous levels. Diuretics are often used in these circumstances, causing the release of sodium and fluid as blood pressure is returned to normal levels. But this treatment just scratches the surface of an insulin disorder that runs very deep. The irony is that even though excess insulin causes fluid retention, diuretics actually stimulate insulin! Crazy isn't it? Save yourself from death by shooting yourself in the head!

2. Hyperinsulinemia alters the mechanics of the blood vessels

In excess, insulin has the power to make arteries less elastic. It also acts as a growth hormone on smooth muscle cells in the walls of the arteries, causing them to increase in thickness, become stiffer and less supple, while at the same time decreasing the volume within the arteries. Is it any wonder blood pressure rises as the heart begins to struggle, forcing blood through these narrow, more rigid arteries?

3. Hyperinsulinemia increases nervous stimulation of the arterial system

The third way insulin causes elevated blood pressure is by raising blood levels of the neurotransmitter norepinephrine. You'll learn a lot about this adrenaline-like substance in a later chapter, it is critical for the formation of memories and heightened states of awareness, yet too much can prevent the laying down of new memories, and can interfere with rational thought and decision making. Just as stress, excitement or intense fear can radically alter your physiological response, it's the adrenaline that causes your heart to beat faster and give you that shaky, uncomfortable feeling. By engaging in habits that over-stimulate insulin, norepinephrine is released into the blood, helping to keep blood pressure high and heart rate above normal. All these factors put unnecessary stress on the heart.

A COMMON TALE OF INSULIN EXCESS

A patient may gain weight and in the process develop high blood pressure. Their doctor may prescribe a mild diuretic and low salt to lower their blood pressure. A few weeks later the patient returns. Their blood pressure has improved but their cholesterol level is elevated (another by-product of insulin excess, as you'll learn shortly). The doctor decides to put the patient on a low fat-high carbohydrate diet, expecting a drop in weight and lowered cholesterol levels, but insulin levels remain high. One month later the patient returns, they're still overweight (due to excess insulin production) with similar cholesterol problems, but this time their tryglycerides or blood sugar levels have increased. If the doctor had looked beyond the symptoms they'd have discovered insulin excess was the root of all the problems.

The actual medications used to regulate blood pressure (Beta-blockers) also stimulate insulin. Can you believe doctors prescribe such drugs to lower blood pressure that actually fuel the original cause? There isn't a medication on the market that lowers insulin, although many stimulate it. Your only chance is to take control of your diet. Let raw foods heal the misery caused by cooked foods and medications.

So there you have it. Insulin excess stimulates high blood pressure in three unique, yet complementary ways. It stimulates the kidneys, causing water retention. This increase in pressure exerts its force on the artery walls, which have been thickened and stripped of their elasticity – again due to insulin. And to top it all off, unbalanced levels of norepinephrine constricts the flow of blood and the pressure heightens. It isn't exactly the ideal way to run your biochemistry is it? With the right use of food, the problem of water retention and high blood pressure can be corrected within a few short weeks. Make sure you use them otherwise…

EXCESS INSULIN CAN PAVE THE WAY
FOR HEART DISEASE

Your heart is immortal if it is supplied with oxygen rich blood via the coronary arteries. If something occludes a coronary artery, compromising blood flow to the heart, such as the formation of plaque, blood can be reduced or cut off completely. The main culprits are cholesterol filled fibrous growths, which may develop on the inner linings of coronary arteries, over a long period of time.

THE DEADLY REALITY OF INSULIN EXCESS

In the early 1960s, Dr Anatolio Cruz and his research team demonstrated the danger of chronically elevated insulin levels. Each day for eight months, they injected insulin into one leg of a large group of dogs. As a control, they injected another leg with a sterile saline solution. The result: No change in the arteries injected with the saline solution, but in the arteries that had been exposed to excess insulin three main developments occurred:

1. The accumulation of cholesterol.
2. The accumulation of fatty acids.
3. Arterial thickening.

Each of these factors compromised blood flow, demonstrating the dangers of engaging in habits that continuously stimulate insulin. The amount of insulin administered to the dogs was relatively small! Can you imagine what happens to individuals who eat and drink in such a way that their bloodstream is never free from insulin? This experiment didn't even last for a year and most people are stimulating excessive amounts of insulin for a lifetime. Take a look at the history books if you haven't yet made the link between recreational food eating (high sugar consumption) and heart disease.

THE INCREASE OF SUGAR CONSUMPTION LEADS
DIRECTLY TO HEART DISEASE

In 1865, human beings consumed about 40 pounds of refined sugar per year and death from cardiovascular disease was extremely rare. By 1900 sugar consumption had risen to 85 pounds per person per year and today it stands at over 120 pounds per person per year. The first heart attack case was not described until 1912. In 1930, heart attacks caused no more that three thousand deaths in the United States. Cardiovascular disease used to kill 1 in 7 people back in the early 1900s but now kills 1 in 2. Are you getting the point?

The occurrence of diabetes has risen at a similar rate, and today accounts for 1 death in 20. Obesity affects about 30% of adults in Western society today, and is highly correlated with cardiovascular disease, diabetes, allergies, cancer, and a host of other ailments. Excessive sugar consumption causes hyperinsulinemia and hyperinsulinemia kills.

HOMOCYSTEINE: VITAMIN DEFICIENCY
AND HEART DISEASE

Homocysteine is produced in the body when the amino acid methionine is metabolised. Usually it is cleared rapidly from your blood before it can damage your arteries. Many heart disease studies point the finger at high levels of homocysteine for the cause of 10% of coronary deaths and a somewhat greater proportion of stroke deaths. This accounts for more than one hundred thousand deaths in the United States every year.

Elevated homocysteine is the result of vitamin deficiency, in particular sub-optimal blood levels of the B complex vitamins, especially folic acid, B6 and/or B12. You need these vitamins to make the enzymes that remove homocysteine efficiently from your body. AFA algae found in E3Live is an excellent source of B vitamins, but remember if you don't eliminate refined sugar, you'll never eliminate the true cause of the problem. Sugar eats away at B vitamins. Eliminate it!

THE HORRIBLE TRUTH ABOUT INSULIN AND
CHOLESTEROL

Imagine knowing more useful facts about cholesterol than the majority of the medical profession. Imagine never having to pop any pills or take any special formulas in order to stabilise your cholesterol within a perfect zone. If you are interested, you need to...

LEARN HOW TO OPERATE YOUR
CHOLESTEROL MANUFACTURING MACHINERY

If you are one of the unfortunate few who have been attempting to lower your cholesterol levels by restricting cholesterol in your diet, you're fighting a losing battle.

Think of how many products you've seen with the infamous words 'cholesterol free' or 'contains no cholesterol'. People don't even know what it is. If you think cholesterol is a fat then you are wrong! It's a pearly white waxy alcohol with a soapy feel. Maybe you've been lead to believe that cholesterol is a deadly killer and leads to heart disease and death. Again, you've been misinformed. As long as you control your cholesterol regulation system, it won't matter if you increase the amount of cholesterol in your diet or decrease it. Your body will adjust accordingly! Concentrating on cholesterol consumption alone could be your biggest downfall, since the cholesterol you eat only accounts for as little as 20% of the total cholesterol in your bloodstream. The other 80% is produced primarily in your liver. It is also produced in your intestines and skin. Each and every cell in your body can make cholesterol, so if you eliminate it from your diet, your liver will produce whatever else is needed to keep your system running smoothly. If you consume large quantities of cholesterol your cell production making machinery will ease up on production.

MANY DOCTORS ARE THROWING
A SPANNER IN THE WORKS!

Many doctors still prescribe a low fat, high carbohydrate diet for lowering dangerously high cholesterol levels, but all this does is stimulate more of the hormone insulin, causing the cells of your body to manufacture more cholesterol. That's the equation: More insulin – More cholesterol synthesis. You'll find out why shortly.

Cholesterol is critical to life, which is why you must learn what it is, where it comes from, how to reduce it (if it is dangerously high) and finally how to control it. You won't have to take any drugs and you certainly won't have to eat a low fat diet. Rather than concentrating on your intake, you'll learn how to control the complex cholesterol regulation system and keep it running smoothly. For now, take a look at the importance of cholesterol. You'll soon discover the endless advantages of keeping blood/cholesterol levels optimal.

◆ Each and every cell in your body requires cholesterol to maintain the structural integrity of its cell membrane. This controls the flow of water and nutrients into the cell and regulates the disposal of waste.

◆ Your brain and central nervous system need cholesterol for normal growth and development and optimal electrical signal transmission. Cholesterol coats the nerves and makes the transmission of nerve impulses possible.

◆ Cholesterol is the building block for many important hormones. For example, the adrenal hormone aldosterone helps to regulate blood pressure, whilst hydrocortisone has a natural steroid type effect. Both are built from cholesterol. The sex hormones (oestrogen and testosterone) are also made from cholesterol.

◆ Your digestion relies heavily on bile acids, especially for the digestion of fats. Cholesterol is the main component of these acids and without it you wouldn't be able to absorb the critical fat-soluble vitamins A, D, E and K.

◆ Cholesterol gives skin its ability to shed water and is a precursor of vitamin D in the skin, essential for protection in the sun.

◆ Tryglycerides allow fat to circulate through the blood and cholesterol plays a major role in this transportation process.

THE SECRET OF CHOLESTEROL CONTROL: KEEPING CHOLESTEROL LEVELS IN A STRICT ZONE

Blood/cholesterol levels may vary from one person to the next, but inside each and every one of your cells, cholesterol levels are always kept in a strict zone. The level of cholesterol within each cell is so important to your health that each one has its own feedback mechanism that informs the cell of the current cholesterol levels. Your bloodstream doesn't possess such a mechanism which explains why the majority of cholesterol problems are due to a build up of plaque within artery walls, rather than a lack of cholesterol at a cellular level.

RESTRICTIVE DIETS, CHOLESTEROL AND CANCER

Very restrictive diets may limit cholesterol intake but more importantly limit the essential nutrients needed for the production of cholesterol. If cells can't take cholesterol from the bloodstream, and the liver is unable to manufacture enough cholesterol, low cell-cholesterol levels cause cells to lose their strength and stability, putting them at risk of infection and malignancy. Rock bottom cholesterol levels can lead to the development of cancer or crippling arthritis.

If you get it right, you can indirectly control cholesterol within the blood and prevent the unnecessary build up of plaque within artery walls, as long as you supply all the necessary nutrients to allow cholesterol formation to continue effortlessly. Let's look in more detail at how you can do this...

REGULATING CHOLESTEROL LEVELS
AND MAINTAINING THE BALANCE

Each and every cell in your body requires a steady supply of cholesterol to sustain health. In order to meet the demands of your cells, cholesterol is supplied in two ways.

1. It's either extracted from the bloodstream, or
2. The cells make their own (or both).

The sensors on the inside of the cells detect the cholesterol level within the cell. If levels fall within the cell, the sensors fire off a series of chemical reactions that cause the cholesterol production line to crank out more cholesterol, or journey to the bloodstream to extract it from the blood. The aim: To restore balance within the cell. This explains why increased levels of cholesterol in the blood can clog the walls of the arteries that supply the heart, body and brain, whilst individual cells are unaffected. As far as individual cells are concerned, the bloodstream is there to supply cholesterol! The cells aren't directly concerned whether levels are too high within the blood. It's up to you to take responsibility of your diet if you want to keep blood-cholesterol levels within a healthy zone. That's where we're headed!

CONTROL THE LOW-DENSITY LIPOPROTEINS (LDLs)

Even though cholesterol occupies your bloodstream, it isn't soluble in your blood. Question: How does it get transported around? Answer: By the lipoproteins. Lipoproteins act like envelopes, encasing cholesterol and tryglycerides allowing them to be transported to the target cells.

There are many varieties of lipoproteins, but for the purpose of this section, concern yourself with only low-density lipoproteins (LDLs). They have been given a bad name since they are known to be the no. 1 villain responsible for developing coronary artery disease. If you can prevent the excessive build up of LDLs in the bloodstream you've got the secret to cholesterol control! Remember, some LDLs are needed to transport linoleic acid into your cells for eicosanoid production.

THE SECRET OF THE LDL RECEPTORS

If a cell is in need of cholesterol, it sends LDL receptors to the surface of the cell, where they lie in wait for cholesterol-filled LDL particles in the blood. When a cholesterol-filled LDL particle passes an LDL receptor, the receptor grabs it and pulls it into the cell. At this point cholesterol has been taken from the blood and transported into the cell where it is needed. Once the LDL receptor has released the LDL particle it heads back to the surface of the cell if more is needed. Blood cholesterol levels are lowered and forces within the cell extract the cholesterol from the LDL particle and utilise the cholesterol for various cellular functions.

If you've had problems with high LDL-blood levels in the past, an increase in these tiny scavengers (LDL receptors) will prevent the excessive build up of LDL cholesterol in your bloodstream, instantly bringing cholesterol into a safe and healthy zone.

THE POWER OF THE LDL RECEPTORS

Researchers discovered that people who develop heart disease in their teens or early twenties have a genetic disorder preventing their cells from making adequate LDL receptors. Thus LDL removal from the blood is incredibly limited causing levels to remain elevated. If LDL levels remain too high for too long, the chances of plaque formation and blockages in coronary arteries increase tremendously. The message: Do whatever you can to ensure that your cells are teeming with the hardworking LDL receptors and you'll keep blood LDLs within the normal range reducing the risk of heart disease.

In fact even if your diet was high in saturated fat and cholesterol, as long as you crank out as many LDL receptors as possible, you could keep your blood cholesterol levels optimal.

MIRACLE MICE CRANK OUT FIVE TIMES MORE LDL RECEPTORS PREVENTING THE PERILS OF HEART DISEASE

Through careful research and experimentation, a group of scientists were able to breed a selection of mice that cranked out five times more LDL receptors in their livers than a control group of mice. The result: The super-mice were able to maintain blood cholesterol levels 50% lower than the mice in the control group.

Even if the researchers fed the mice diets high in saturated fat and cholesterol, the LDL values in the control group went through the roof, whilst the super-mice maintained normal LDL levels similar to the previous diet.

THE SECRET: INCREASE THE PRODUCTION OF THE LDL RECEPTORS AND WAVE GOOD-BYE TO CHOLESTEROL PROBLEMS ONCE AND FOR ALL!

The trick to increasing LDL receptor production is to limit cholesterol production inside the cells. That way it is inevitable that the cell would have no other option than to increase the number of LDL receptors and send them to the cell surface to scavenge cholesterol from the blood. It may come as no surprise that a drug exists to do just that. Its name is lovastatin (Mevacor) and it is an incredibly potent cholesterol-lowering drug. The reason it is so successful is because it slows down the activity of an enzyme known as 3-hydroxy-3-methylglutaryl-coenzyme A reductase (HMG-CoA reductase). Now there's a mouthful!

LIMIT HMG-CoA REDUCTASE AND YOU HAVE THE ANSWER TO YOUR CHOLESTEROL LOWERING PRAYERS

If you limit the production of this enzyme, you reduce cholesterol synthesis inside of each cell. Less cholesterol synthesis forces the cell to manufacture more LDL receptors, which scavenge LDLs from the blood and thus deliver cholesterol to the cells. As with many powerful drugs you can expect side effects! The term 'side-effect' is a term used by the medical profession to hide the truth. What they really mean is 'toxic-effects'. 'Side-effects' presuppose the primary effects are beneficial. All drugs, medicines, pills and potions are poisons. Rashes, muscular disorders, liver problems, gallbladder disorders and psychiatric disturbances are hardly just 'side effects'. They are poisonous toxic effects of a substance your body tries desperately to eliminate. So how do you limit the production of HMG-CoA reductase without drugs?

THE MASTER HORMONES OF
ENERGY METABOLISM ARE BACK!

Two hormones determine the activity of the enzyme HMG-CoA reductase – insulin and glucagon. Insulin stimulates HMG-CoA reductase. Glucagon inhibits it. Insulin is the key to increased cellular cholesterol, basically killing any chances of maintaining healthy blood cholesterol levels.

Glucagon inhibits the activity of HMG-CoA and as a result is just as powerful as lovastatin. Increase glucagon and you decrease the cholesterol producing machinery inside the cells, forcing LDL receptors to rush to the cell surface in an effort to pull cholesterol from the blood, restoring the appropriate balance.

REDUCE INSULIN AND
SILENCE CHOLESTEROL PRODUCTION

Insulin speeds up the workers within the cholesterol manufacturing pipeline, leading to a build up and surplus within each cell. At this point there is no need for the cell to retrieve any from the bloodstream and hey presto, as if like magic, cholesterol begins to build up in the blood. If you want potentially life threatening levels of cholesterol in your blood, increase your insulin levels.

Reduce insulin and immediately the signal that causes an increase in cholesterol synthesis is silenced and the cells begin to harvest the necessary cholesterol directly from the blood, causing blood levels to drop. Even if your diet was rich in red meats, egg yolk, cheese, butter and cream, as long as you keep insulin and glucagon balanced, you'll maintain healthy cholesterol levels, somewhere between 180 to

200mg/dl. Your LDL/HDL ratio will be under 3 and any extra fat will simply raise levels of HDLs (high-density lipoproteins). LDLs have a reputation for causing ill health because they are the main culprits in the development of coronary artery disease. HDLs have a reputation for being 'good' because they scavenge cholesterol from the tissues, including the lining of the coronary arteries, and transport it back to the cells of the liver where it is disposed of.

PARAMETERS OF CHOLESTEROL SUCCESS

Your risk of heart disease increases if LDL levels are above normal. But the real key to optimal cholesterol levels is keeping an eye on these parameters.

1. Total cholesterol divided by HDL should be below 4.
2. LDL divided by HDL should be below 3.
3. Total cholesterol should be kept between 180-200mg/dl range.

As blood cholesterol levels rise, so do your chances for heart disease. As blood cholesterol levels fall, cell cholesterol levels can drop to dangerous levels, increasing your chances of cerebral haemorrhage, gallbladder disease and cancer. Nutrient deficiencies can lead to sub-optimal manufacture of cholesterol, so eat a wide variety of life-enhancing raw plant foods and take control of the insulin/glucagon balancing act. Your health is at risk if you don't.

THE DEADLY POTENTIAL OF REFINED SUGAR

Sugar is the enemy! It over-stimulates insulin causing biochemical destruction whilst stripping your body of vital nutrients and destroying any chance of perfect health. Memorise the following list:

1. Refined sugar interferes with the function of essential fatty acids.
2. Refined sugar promotes bacterial invasion, as in rheumatism, inflammation of the heart and the more publicised tooth decay.
3. Refined sugar feeds bacteria, yeast, fungus, and cancer cells.
4. Refined sugar prevents the body from absorbing calcium. It also pulls calcium, chromium and other minerals from the body.

5. Refined sugar interferes with vitamin C transport and therefore with immune function (The colds we get right after Christmas? They're from eating chocolate, sweets, and cake and from drinking too much alcohol, all of which are full of sugar!)

6. If refined sugar is consumed just before bedtime, it destroys the body's immune system's ability to build antibodies, which normally occurs an hour and a half into sleep.

7. Refined sugar may, during the filtering process, have carcinogenic impurities introduced into it.

8. Refined sugar plays havoc with blood sugar levels by raising them temporarily and then lowering them to dangerous levels if they cannot be stored.

9. Refined sugar prevents B complex vitamins and other nutrients from being absorbed.

10. Refined sugar is speculated as being a leading cause of headaches.

11. Refined sugar causes fermentation within the alimentary canal.

12. Refined sugar produces an acid that etches the protective tooth enamel and fosters gum disease.

13. Refined sugar interferes with insulin function causing the pancreas to produce excess amounts of insulin.

14. Refined sugar can increase adrenaline production by up to four times, making it a very powerful internal stressor.

15. Refined sugar is physically habit forming. It has been theorised that the addiction to refined sugar, which begins in youth, is the basis of all addictive behaviour lasting throughout a lifetime.

16. Refined sugar doesn't satisfy hunger and creates a craving for more.

17. Refined sugar cross-links proteins and speeds up ageing.

18. As little as six teaspoons of sugar a day can suppress the immune system by up to 25%, with the suppressing effect beginning almost immediately and lasting for up to five hours. How easy is it to eat six teaspoons? Very easy! One chocolate bar would be enough. A 12oz can of cola contains nine teaspoons. Eliminate sugar!

FREE YOURSELF FROM HYPERINSULINEMIA
FREE YOURSELF FROM AN EARLY GRAVE

So there you have it! Hyperinsulinemia is the primary cause of obesity, diabetes, fluid retention, high blood pressure, unfavourable cholesterol levels and heart disease. The message: Keep insulin under constant control by eating powerful nutrient rich raw plant foods. Education gives you the knowledge to make decisions with confidence. Take what you've learned and do what most doctors fail to do – take control of the underlying problem of hyperinsulinemia and listen to the silence as the messages of detrimental health (obesity, diabetes, hypertension, problematical cholesterol and heart disease) begin to fade away.

THE RAW PERFECTION EVALUATION:
Do you realise how detrimental excess insulin production can be to optimal health?
Are you doing everything in your power to control insulin production with the foods you eat?

Having built an aerobic base, it's important you use anaerobic exercise (weights and resistance training) to unleash a cascade of youth enhancing hormones on your body. With time and effort you'll slow down the ageing process and give yourself a greater chance of longevity...

CHAPTER 10

EXERCISE:
THE CHAMPION HORMONAL
REGULATOR

If you arrive at the gym and push yourself to the limit, only to find yourself tired and listless, pay close attention, you could be doing yourself more harm than good! But fear not! You're about to learn a variety of principles on the cutting edge of health and fitness.

Many people struggle with their fitness because they've been conditioned to think NO PAIN – NO GAIN! They spend maybe 60 – 90 minutes pushing themselves to the limit in an effort to burn as many calories as possible, not realising that the calorie content of their next meal will probably replace what they've just burned up! It's not the calories you want to be concerned with, it's the hormonal cascade you set in motion before and after you exercise that determines whether you benefit or not. This is where food steps in! As I've said before, focusing on calorie expenditure is about as futile as eating a big plate of pasta before you exercise, aggravating insulin output, and expecting to be full of energy. Forget about counting calories and learn to apply the following distinctions. If you do, you'll experience metabolic freedom as you learn how to *burn* fat as your primary fuel.

PEOPLE ARE ONLY BEGINNING TO LEARN ABOUT THE POWER OF HORMONAL CONTROL

When I started out as a fitness instructor, if someone had approached me, and asked me about the hormonal effects of exercise, I would have struggled to make up an answer! Even to this day, many nutritionists have little or no idea of the effects food and exercise has on hormonal control. Hopefully, if you've read this book from cover to cover, you'll realise that food is your No.1 modulator of hormones, but exercise also plays a critical role. Exercise increases your control over insulin, helping you to burn more fat, whilst stimulating a number of hormones that slow down the ageing process. It's up to you to...

CHOOSE THE BEST FUEL FOR THE TASK AT HAND

You may think that carbohydrate is the best source of energy for your muscles, but you couldn't be further from the truth! The most efficient source of energy is fat. It is more plentiful, and supplies more than twice the energy of carbohydrates. The important point to remember is this: When you exercise the enzymes present in the mitochondria (factories of the cell) use the raw materials of carbohydrate or fat to replenish the supplies of ATP (adenosine triphosphate) needed for muscle contraction. No ATP – No muscle contraction! What do you think is more efficient at replenishing these supplies? The answer: FAT! It's up to you to gear your body towards the release of fat to maximise your body's potential. So how do you access it? By eating foods that keep the balance between insulin and glucagon favourable, optimising eicosanoid production. This advice isn't new to you but what follows is. Welcome to...

YOUR THREE WINDOWS OF OPPORTUNITY

If you want to maximise every workout, simply follow these three steps. They are incredibly powerful and once you've experimented with them, you'll understand why!

♦ If you were to look at a clock, 30 – 45 minutes before you start to exercise, what would the time be? This time is critical because it is where you'll apply your first hormonal distinction. At this time, your muscles are relatively relaxed and are putting minimal stress on blood glucose levels. As you begin to workout your blood glucose levels begin to drop, allowing glucagon to exert its power. Glucagon, as you'll remember, is the hormone primarily responsible for keeping your blood glucose levels tightly controlled. If insulin is too high, glucagon will be inhibited.

In order to stimulate glucagon 30 to 45 minutes before a workout, eat a portion of high quality organic greens/wheatgrass juice/E3Live with some raw plant fat (coconut water), and ensure the portion is very small. If you concentrate on eating foods high in the amino acid tyrosine, such as soy foods, you'll also stimulate the energising neurotransmitter dopamine. Your hormones will now orchestrate themselves so that you release maximum energy during your workout and burn fat as your primary fuel.

♦ As soon as you complete your workout, your insulin levels will be quite low. Now, although this is favourable, the problem is that having been depressed during exercise, they begin to automatically increase. If insulin rises too high, growth hormone becomes inhibited. In this second window of opportunity, a similar snack with greens and raw plant fats will prepare your body for the maximum release of growth hormone that is released 15 to 30 minutes after you finish your anaerobic workout. (Nuts and seeds are plentiful in the amino acid arginine that also stimulate growth hormone.)

♦ Since demands on the body have increased during exercise, muscle cells need to be fully replenished. The best way to accomplish this is to ensure that in the third window of opportunity you eat minimal amounts of sugary fruits, but plenty of raw greens/wheatgrass juice/E3Live, whilst supplying a quality source of raw plant fats. If you are going to accompany your choice of foods with fruits or vegetables, ensure they are of the non-stimulating variety. See the last few pages of chapter 8 – Eicosanoids. The fat will slow the rate of carbohydrates into your bloodstream, leaving your meal complete. This final window lasts from the time you finish exercising for about another 2 hours. Again, by keeping the portion relatively small, minimal energy will be spent on digestion. This combination of greens and fats is far more superior than trying to replenish your muscle supplies with carbohydrates alone. It is also a combination that allows you to...

ENERGISE YOUR BLOOD AND BUILD A POWERFUL BODY

An excellent formula for energising the blood and building a powerful body involves the use of young coconut water and freshly made green juice. If you are a body builder or an athlete, this formula is a must! Young coconut water and green juice directly targets the blood. Here's why:

1. In the plant world young fresh coconut water is virtually identical in structure to human blood plasma, which makes up 55% of your blood. It is also the highest source of natural electrolytes (electrically conductive charged minerals in solution that directly nourish the tissues).
2. Chlorophyll found in green juice, is the closest substance to human haemoglobin in the plant world.

Put these two together and you have the ultimate blood building/revitalising formula. Remember the Golden Rule: When you rebuild your blood you rebuild your body.

By drinking up to four coconuts worth of young coconut water daily you'll build exceptional health and strength. Make sure you scoop out the pulp and use it to make 'milkshake style' smoothies! When it comes to foods as powerful as young coconuts, if you throw out the pulp you'll miss out on one of natures finest gifts.

Another food that provides particularly excellent benefits is raw coconut butter (oil), it is easily digested and excellent for people who have trouble digesting fats. Coconut oil consists of 48% lauric acid, a substance that exhibits anti-microbial, anti-bacterial, and anti-fungal properties.

Coconuts are an excellent source of raw plant fat, necessary to lubricate the digestive tract. They also deliver specific protection to cell walls. Raw fats also deliver extra electrons to the cells, proving to be excellent anti-oxidants. The best coconuts are young coconuts. You'll recognise them because they are white on the outside or green if uncut. The brown hairy ones are old and dry.

BECOMING ONE OF THE
STRONGEST ANIMALS ON EARTH

The gorilla, the elephant, the hippopotamus, the giraffe, the rhinoceros, the horse, the bull, the buffalo, etc. stand head and shoulders above the rest of the animal kingdom when it comes to raw strength. If you want to develop strength like them, you have to eat like them! What do you think the largest and strongest mammals on Earth eat? 100% raw plant food! If a gorilla can bench-press the equivalent of 4000lbs, what magical process allows him to build muscle without eating animal protein? Answer: There is no rule. If a gorilla is able to synthesise proteins from raw plant foods, so can you!

TWO CRITICAL COMPONENTS FOR BUILDING
UNRIVALLED STRENGTH

Think of fat as the delivery vehicle and green leafy vegetables as the provider of the minerals necessary for exceptional muscle and bone development. If either of these are missing, health will be compromised. Use fat strategically and you'll build an all-powerful physique. Remember coconuts, avocados, olives or nuts are great for this purpose. Olives are one of the best bodybuilding foods on the planet. For a vitamin/mineral boost, choose freshly made juices from fruits and vegetables that overflow with Nature's bounty. Pills and artificially created powders will not build RAW HEALTH.

LIMIT ALL INSULIN STIMULATING FOODS AND
MAXIMISE RAW PLANT FATS AND GREENS

The master formula for gaining strength and weight on an all-raw diet is to begin by limiting sweet fruits and replacing them with non-sweet fruits, and ensuring the majority of your diet is plentiful in green leafed vegetables and plant fats. A great combination for weight gain is to eat avocados and olives and chase them with fresh green juice.

INCREDIBLE STRENGTH, INCREDIBLE POWER, NATURAL MEASURES

The gorilla is the strongest land mammal pound for pound and all it does is eat in alignment with nature. It doesn't sit down to a juicy steak every evening or eat eggs for breakfast. Do you really think if a gorilla ate bread, meat, cheese, chocolate, crisps etc. it would possess such strength? The answer is obvious!

The protein theory essentially states that you *need* flesh protein to build healthy flesh protein. The raw food facts say this is one of the biggest lies ever told and if it were true, then gorillas should have to eat flesh to develop their incredibly muscular 400+ pound (180kg) bodies.

The gorilla eats nearly 80% green leafed vegetation and fruit. Celery (the favourite of the gorilla) should be eaten and/or juiced often to provide the sodium necessary to balance out the high potassium content of fruit. I'll repeat, the gorilla, zebra, giraffe, hippo, rhino, or elephant build their enormous musculature on green leafy vegetation. The cow carries in excess of 1,000 pounds (450kg) of protein flesh, and all it eats is grass. Every amino acid can be found in grass, which is why a cow can build such an enormous powerful body. You would look ridiculous grazing out in a field for days at a time, but you can begin to increase your consumption of fresh raw greens. Simple.

FOUNTAIN OF YOUTH BREAKTHROUGH

In a moment you are going to read about a substance that has amazing effects on your body, well-being and health. It's also a substance that has been documented in many journals related to the slowing of the ageing process. I'll call it substance X and later will reveal its true identity.

In 1990, The New England Journal of Medicine produced a very interesting report. Daniel Rudman, M. D., and his research group at the Medical College of Wisconsin produced some amazing results when they injected substance X in a group of elderly males. Dr. Rudman's group showed that tiny amounts of substance X injected just beneath the skin of 61-81 year-old males produced almost unbelievable results in less than six months. They reported that:

♦ Lean body mass increased by 8.8%.
♦ Body fat decreased by 14.4%.
♦ Bone density increased in the lumbar spinal bones.
♦ Skin thickness increased by 7.1% (thin, brittle skin is one of the consequences of ageing).

All these changes were a result of the subjects artificially increasing the quantity of substance X in their body (the subjects didn't change their diet or exercise) and after only six months of therapy with minuscule amounts of this extremely potent substance the results were amazing. In Dr Rudmens words, "The changes were equivalent in magnitude to the changes incurred during 10 to 20 years of reverse ageing."

Even many clinics have begun popping up all over Mexico and other less medically regulated countries which administer substance X.

HAVE I GOT YOUR ATTENTION?

Do you want to know what substance X is? Of course you do! But first, let me give you another example of how powerful it really is, before I share with you the secret to producing more of it in your body naturally.

A study performed at the University of New Mexico, demonstrated that in a six week period, weight lifters injected with substance X lost four times more body fat, and gained four times more lean body mass, compared to those who received only a placebo. Injections of substance X are a difficult and dangerous way to trim fat and build muscle, and are only used to treat unusually small children under medical supervision. Any other use is illegal; the side effects can be very destructive. People who do inject substance X increase their body's chances of shutting down its natural release, increasing the chances of diabetes!

Well you've waited long enough. Substance X – the fountain of youth – is human growth hormone (HGH). It is a profound tissue building (anabolic) hormone produced in the pituitary gland (a small gland located at the base of the skull) and is secreted at intervals throughout the day. HGH stimulates tissue growth, increases muscle tone and lean mass, enhances flexibility, thickens muscles, stimulates the growth of bones and organs, mobilises fat stores, shifts the metabolism to the preferential use of fat, and helps maintain healthy tissues. Forget injections to increase HGH levels...

USE EXERCISE AND ACCESS
THE FOUNTAIN OF YOUTH NATURALLY

By exercising anaerobically you can naturally and powerfully release more of this substance, building muscle and burning fat in the process. Start by lifting light weights until you are comfortable with the movements and then increase from there. Take a look at the body of a world class sprinter, conditioned swimmer or professional body builder. Their lean, toned bodies highlight the remarkable effect of anaerobic training. Growth hormone fosters a regeneration of youth.

HOW DO YOU CONTROL YOUR PHYSIOLOGY
TO MAXIMISE THE RELEASE OF GROWTH HORMONE

Teenagers release a lot of growth hormone naturally and can eat a lot of 'junk food' without affecting its production. Blood samples show that the older you are the less growth hormone you produce. HGH is released into your blood stream at two specific times.

♦ About 90 minutes after you go to sleep, and
♦ Once before you wake-up in the morning.

High levels of HGH naturally drop over time. By age sixty, about 30 % of men produce little or none of the substance. It is assumed that women continue to secrete growth hormone into their old age, and thus live longer.

IT DOESN'T HAVE TO BE LIKE THIS

The reason adults don't produce as much as adolescents, isn't because they can't, but because they are more sensitive to the factors that prevent its release. The potential is present in all of us to release more HGH into the bloodstream given the optimal environment, and guess what controls the release of human growth hormone from the pituitary gland? Good eicosanoids. Here's a list of the factors that stimulate the release of growth hormone:

♦ Decreased blood glucose levels.
♦ Foods rich in the amino acid arginine – nuts and seeds.

- Carbohydrate restricted diet.
- Fasting.
- Increased protein diet.
- Free fatty acid decrease.
- PGE1 (a good eicosanoid).
- Stage 4 sleep.
- Exercise.

As you can see, if you follow all the principles of RAW PERFECTION, you'll be indirectly increasing your chances of maximally stimulating HGH anyway!

BECOME A LOVING PARENT
AND NUTURE YOUR NEWBORN

If new born babies are touched and caressed, their levels of growth hormone increase and the protective coating of the motor nerves (myelin sheath) becomes thicker. A mother's loving urge to cuddle her baby translates directly into life-sustaining biochemical reactions. Babies deprived of loving attention can become emotionally stunted or dysfunctional.

A GOOD NIGHT'S SLEEP IS CRITICAL

Growth hormone is secreted in a pulsatile surge during stage 3 and 4 sleep, just prior to REM (Rapid Eye Movement – the first hour or two after reaching deep sleep.) In this time period your body repairs itself for the next day of operation. The better your quality of sleep, the more growth hormone you'll release.

One simple strategy you can adopt if you want to increase your chances of releasing a maximum surge of HGH during sleep is to eat an insulin controlling, glucagon-stimulating snack an hour before you retire. A carbohydrate rich snack will raise your insulin levels and *inhibit* the release of HGH from the pituitary gland.

You may think these principles are restrictive and in a sense you are right! They are about fine-tuning. Don't expect to master them straightaway, give yourself a day or a week or however long you need before you are committed to excellence. Remember by continually fine-tuning your habits, you decrease your chances of going back to bad ones. That's the secret! As I've said earlier, my worse days nutritionally are better than most people's best!

ANAEROBIC EXERCISE RELEASES
A POWERFUL SHOT OF GROWTH HORMONE

When you begin working out with dumbbells or resistance machines, if you exercise at 80% or more of your capacity, you engage your body's fat-burning metabolism, sending it into overdrive. The effects don't just last whilst you are training hard, but last for many hours after you've finished. Simply enlist the help of a gym instructor or contact www.rawperfection.co.uk for information on personal training. With the addition of three fifteen-minute weekly resistance-training sessions, it won't be long before you see incredible results. If you need to lose unwanted fat then this principle alone will help stoke the fire of your fat burning metabolism by increasing the density of your muscles.

♦ A long-term study of 17300 Harvard alumni, published in the New England Journal of Medicine, concluded that intense exercise could add years to your life and life to your years. It showed that people who participated in intense exercise lived the longest.

The aim here is to stack the deck. If you add one principle onto the next, over and over again, you gradually build a foundation for extraordinary health, people will look at you with awe and respect as you begin to look and feel better than ever before. Gradually what was once hard will seem easy.

YOU ARE ALWAYS YOUNG ENOUGH
TO START LIFTING WEIGHTS

Laboratory tests in Miami, Florida have produced exciting results. People in their sixties who've spent at least ten to fifteen years with minimal muscle tone are learning to lift weights and create muscle mass equivalent to that of twenty-one-year-olds, with energy levels to match. Yes! You can be as strong in your seventies and eighties as you were in your twenties and thirties! Think of HGH as one of the most powerful fat-burning hormones in your body. Fat burning takes place in the mitochondria of muscle cells. The more muscle you have, the more of these little energy factories you have, increasing your fat-burning potential. It's that simple. When someone's metabolism slows right down, they reduce their ability to lose weight. Don't let this be you! Use the power of anaerobic exercise to increase your muscle density, strengthen your bones and speed up your metabolism.

WARNING: WEIGHT-BEARING EXERCISE INCREASES BONE DENSITY – BUT NOT WITHOUT A GOOD DIET

Any horse vet will tell you, if you want to kill a horse, keep it locked up in a stable! Most vets know that if you let it get out and run around, it will probably get better. The fastest way to kill a senior citizen is to do the same – trap them in room or a home where movement is limited.

According to Dr Robert Schulze, a daily walk of 45 mins can cause dramatic increases in bone density. But to build bone, your bone cells also need nutrition. Weight-bearing exercise will increase your bone density, as long as the necessary raw materials are present within the body to begin with. Without quality nutrition, it doesn't matter how much exercise you do, you're just going to build brittle bone, or no bone at all.

Bone cells will not grow bone from processed junk food or soft drinks. These foods have been shown to degenerate and eliminate all the usable calcium from the body. If you are 50 years old and showing signs of osteoporosis/low bone density – weight bearing exercises may actually increase your chances of a fracture. The worst mistake you can make is look towards milk for stronger bones.

THE PERILS OF PASTEURISATION

Many people still think of pasteurisation as one of the most important discoveries of the 20th Century, but a study in the British Medical Journal (Vol. 14, No. 10) written in 1960 clearly highlights the dangers of pasteurisation. Entitled…

'The Effect of Heat Treatment on the Nutritive Value of Milk for the Young Calf: The effect of Ultra-High Temperature Treatment and of Pasteurisation'

In this study, researchers fed a group of calves their mother's milk, after it had been cooked, and in nine out of ten cases the calf died before reaching maturity. Can you believe this? Can you believe advertisers spend millions in an effort to convince us it is a near perfect food! It can't even sustain life in the animal it was designed for, how is it supposed to help you build health?! Conclusion: Cooked milk is a poison. Science has proved it. What does your common sense tell you? Think about it!

The dairy council advises children to drink lots of milk to grow up big and strong. What they don't tell you is the enzyme necessary for the digestion of milk is lactase, and 20% of Caucasian children and 80% of black children have no lactase in their intestines.

INCREASE YOUR BONE DENSITY WITH SUPER-NUTRIENT NON-DAIRY FOODS ...AND LET THE X-RAYS PROVE IT!

Medical Herbalist Dr Richard Schulz, renowned for his success with so-called impossible patients, used carrot juice regularly with his patients to build strong bones, especially if they were calcium deficient. Take a look at these figures and you'll see why.

♦ An 8-oz. glass of fortified milk has about 250 mg of calcium – with a very low assimilation percentage.
♦ An 8-oz. glass of carrot juice has 100-400 mg of calcium (depending on the quality of the carrots), and you'll assimilate all the calcium!

Many of Dr Schulze's patients were able to dramatically increase their own bone density, from the simple inclusion of a few daily glasses of fresh carrot juice and other naturally high calcium foods, without calcium tablets.

One lady he treated sustained severe injuries after a nasty fall. She broke a wrist on one hand, her elbow on the other, and also fractured her hip! Doctors tested her bone density and were so concerned about the frailty of her bones, they wanted to put steel pins in her limbs in case of future accidents. The lady refused the operations and decided she wanted the bones to heal. She consulted Dr Schulze who put her on a program of increased exercise, and a diet of fresh juices high in calcium, whilst reducing protein.

If you mix green leafy vegetables such as parsley, kale and chard with a carrot juice base, your calcium intake will skyrocket. Add some nuts or an avocado, to slow the release of the sugar from the carrots into the bloodstream (carrots are hybrid foods) and you're on your way to RAW PERFECTION! Sea vegetables such as seaweed and kelp are also an excellent source of calcium, as is AFA algae found in E3Live. Sesame seeds are another food source often underestimated for their potent calcium content. Anyway...

WHAT HAPPENED TO THE LADY?

After following the program for two months, with no hormone replacement or calcium tablets, her bone density was checked again. The doctors' jaws dropped in amazement! The bone X-rays in front of them looked no different than those of a teenager! The message: Use quality nutrition and expect to be rewarded in more ways than one. Back to the chase. Start lifting weights and watch in awe as you...

TURN YOUR BODY INTO A FAT BURNING FURNACE

Weight training also stimulates the release of the hormone testosterone. This can be viewed as growth hormone's comrade in arms and is a vital element in muscular development, helping to build a larger fat burning potential.

Testosterone is also an aphrodisiac, increasing libido in both males and females. When you train with weights, ensure you only have very short rest periods between sets (approximately 25 – 60 seconds). By doing so you'll more easily keep the intensity of your workout higher and thus stimulate both HGH and testosterone. Loss of muscle mass/strength is the primary cause of loss of functionality in later life. This kind of training represents your best insurance policy.

Relaxation and rest are both critical in triggering large quantities of both HGH and testosterone. In fact professional body builders such as Frank Zane use mind machines immediately after a workout to promote the release of these powerful youth enhancing hormones. See chapter 12 – The Electrifying Power Of Mind Technology to learn more about these amazing peak performance/relaxation tools.

STRESS INTERFERES WITH TESTOSTERONE PRODUCTION:
THE PERILS OF OVER TRAINING

Anaerobic training stresses your body a lot more than aerobic training. Whether you're a seasoned body builder or just starting out, remember one thing – after approximately 45 minutes of weight lifting, cortisol levels increase so much, any more training is detrimental to your health. Most of the negative effects of over-training can be attributed to excess cortisol production, increased Interleukin-6 production and a decrease in DHEA. Professor Patrick Bouic, co-author of 'The Immune System Cure' and other researchers have discovered that the function of the T-cells (the generals of our immune army) and natural killer cells (our cancer fighting cells) is suppressed by over-training. In addition, testosterone levels begin to drop as more precursors (building blocks) of testosterone are diverted to facilitate increased cortisol production in response to exercise-related stress. Testosterone is anabolic, building strength and health. Cortisol is catabolic and breaks down tissue, running you down. The more you reduce excess cortisol, the greater your chance of unleashing the anabolic benefits of testosterone.

I'll make the point clear, professional bodybuilders usually train more intensely for shorter periods of time and keep the rest time between sets as low as 25 seconds. You may not be able to lift as much weight, but by keeping the training intensity high, muscle growth will occur at an accelerated rate. Keep the balance between exercising and rest! Your health is at risk if you don't!

RELAX LADIES! YOU'RE NOT GOING TO LOOK LIKE
ARNOLD SCHWARZENEGGER!

Ladies. If you don't want to build a body like Arnold Schwarzenegger, take a deep breath and relax. Fortunately your female hormones will prevent you from piling on the pounds, and your lack of male hormones will keep you slim (even if you train extensively). Anabolic steroids make professional women body builders look like men. Even if you train hard, you'll simply replace intra-muscular fat with muscle, making your muscles not larger but denser, increasing your fat burning metabolic potential. Not only will you look better, but you'll have built a bigger dumping ground for blood sugar, causing your body to store less fat.

Everett Smith, director of biogerontology laboratories at the University of Wisconsin, reported in 1993 that a group of middle-aged women, who did nothing more than hoist 5-pound weights, once a week for over four years, slowed the loss of bone mass in their arms by a staggering 50%.

A loss of bone mass is one of the leading causes of fractures in the elderly, particularly in women after the onset of the menopause. In worst cases, bones are so weak that the act of stepping off a high curb can lead to fracture. Every year, 1000s of elderly people die from the complications following hip fractures. Use resistance training to your advantage and...

BANISH THE INHIBITORS OF GROWTH HORMONE

As with almost every system in the body, there are two sides to the story. Just as a number of factors stimulate the pituitary gland to release growth hormone, other factors inhibit its release. Take a look at the list and prepare to fine-tune your understanding even more.

Factors that inhibit the release of growth hormone
♦ Increased blood glucose levels.
♦ Increased blood free fatty acids.
♦ Obesity.
♦ Pregnancy.

People who eat sweet, starchy, or otherwise carbohydrate laden foods before they go to bed, inhibit the normal shot of growth hormone released an hour or so after falling asleep. If you choose to eat fruit, choose from grapefruits, apples, pears, cherries, peaches as they are low on the glycemic index. The same principle is true for people who either eat high carbohydrate foods before or immediately after a workout. The pulse of growth hormone released through exercise generally hits the circulation towards the end of the workout and immediately after. To inhibit this growth hormone surge, people only have to eat a power bar, chocolate bar or hybrid food, or drink a fizzy sports/soft drink.

Excess insulin in your blood stream is the main cause of the problem. If insulin levels are up, growth hormone levels are down, whether you've trained well or not. If you are smart, you'll steer clear of the high-carbohydrate energy drinks – before, during, and after exercise!

Many fitness instructors still advise these kinds of foods claiming they give you "explosive, high carbohydrate energy." Scientific fact states that all they do is raise your insulin levels and inhibit the release of HGH.

THE PERILS OF CONVENTIONAL BODY BUILDING HABITS

In an effort to maximise weight gain, conventional bodybuilders usually eat all day long, but by eating all day (5 or 6 big meals plus shakes and snacks) the metabolism begins to run at an accelerated rate, decreasing recovery time and increasing the need for sleep. The energy spent on digestion, assimilation, and elimination is enormous. Is there an alternative?

SUMO WRESTLERS AND RAPID WEIGHT GAIN

Extra-ordinary goals require extra-ordinary measures. One type of weight gain strategy that may be useful is similar to the one used by Sumo wrestlers. Although they eat cooked food, and are incredibly fat, their method is intriguing. Sumo wrestlers fast all day, but right before they go to bed; they eat an enormous cooked meal. Throughout the day the body responds by 'thinking' there's a shortage of food and goes into a starvation/scarcity/storage mode, conserving energy, whilst the metabolism slows. With the metabolism slowed, the body isn't ready for the massive intake of food right before bedtime. It fails to process and assimilate the majority of it and unhealthy weight gain is the result.

I wouldn't recommend this strategy to anyone, other than those who wish to gain strength and muscle mass at the expense of health. Eat large meals when you do eat and ensure the foods you eat are made from the finest raw plant fats and green leafy vegetables.

Once your ideal weight is gained, you can return to a more sustainable eating schedule. Raw foodists who eat all day are generally thin. When your body thinks there is an abundance of food, your metabolism speeds up in order to process the sustained food intake. The grazing rather than gorging strategy is one of the best for those who want to lose weight. However, if you want to gain weight, concentrate your focus on green leafy vegetables and fats primarily.

By eating raw and consuming significant amounts of green-leafy vegetable juice (16-24 ounces daily), recovery time can be decreased dramatically.

RAW BODYBUILDERS PAVE THE WAY FOR TRUE HEALTH

Stephen Arlin, author of Raw Power and keen body builder lost 51 pounds when he decided to embrace the 100% raw food lifestyle dropping from 238lbs to 187lbs at 6'2". That's detoxification for you! He then gained 40lbs back through hard work and discipline at the gym. He now weighs in at 225lbs. By weight, his diet consists of 60% raw, organic fruit, 30% raw, organic, green leafy vegetables, and 10% raw organic nuts and sunflower seeds. Yes, you will lose weight on a 100% raw diet, but it will be unhealthy weight, and yes with hard work and commitment you'll build an even stronger body, capable of incredible achievements! Let Stephen Arlin be a source of inspiration and buy his book from www.rawfood.com!

GAIN WEIGHT BY ABSORBING MORE NUTRIENTS

Total health is a personal adventure! By simply increasing the amount of raw food in your diet you can revolutionise your health! There are, however, many other avenues to fine-tune your health. One problem people encounter without knowing it is the inability to absorb nutrients due to an encrusted intestinal tract. Whether you want to gain weight/lose weight or just increase your health you must increase your ability to absorb nutrients. A total raw food diet will eventually dislodge encrusted mucus from the intestinal wall and gradually enhance food absorption. An excellent way to enhance the process and accelerate the removal of this debris is by a series of colon irrigations (6-10) and a herbal cleanse program. Go to www.fresh-network.com for more information on both.

Parasitic infections within the system can cause emaciation and prevent the gaining of weight. The best way to prevent this from happening is again by having a series of colonics and by including garlic, onions, hot peppers, ginger, and spicy wild greens (wild mustard is excellent) in your diet. These foods will burn out a parasitic infection.

WARNING: IF YOU ARE STILL GOING TO EAT MEAT – TAKE NOTE!

Animal protein leaves behind the end products uric acid and urea, which if not eliminated thoroughly can prove to be very harmful. If you haven't yet decided to gradually switch to a 100% raw diet, then minimise animal flesh and dairy products and accompany them with green leafed vegetables which alkalise your system. Meat protein acidifies, but by including an abundance of greens, you can put up a good fight. The fibre in the greens will help push everything through the digestive system efficiently.

Natural sources of fat, such as nuts, seeds and avocados are phosphorus-residue foods. Your body won't absorb their fat as easily unless you combine them with enough calcium-residue foods, such as green leafy vegetables. Nuts with green leafy vegetables provide an acid-alkaline balance for excellent body building purposes. Nuts are acidic – EAT THEM IN VERY SMALL QUANTITIES. For every 10g of nuts eaten, eat/blend/juice 100g green leafy vegetables.

MINERAL DEPLETION: THE DANGERS OF PUSHING THE LIMITS

Have you ever heard of professional athletes dropping dead on the sports field? According to the Centre for Disease Control in Atlanta, 100,000 youngsters/sports professionals die each year from cardiovascular disorders. Almost half of this number played basketball. The intensity of basketball causes players to sweat profusely leading to the loss of many vital nutrients, which if not replaced, can eventually lead to chronic deficiency and maybe even death.

If you think a simple sports drink will replace nutrients lost during exertion, then think again! The majority of sports drinks are loaded with salt, potassium, food colouring and sugar, further depleting valuable minerals and upsetting the acid/alkaline balance.

Healthy blood falls into a very narrow range on the pH scale between 7.3 and 7.45. This may not appear to be a big difference, but in terms of oxygen content, tenths and hundredths of a point make a huge difference. Blood with a pH of 7.45 contains 64.7% more oxygen than blood with a pH of 7.3. Values above or below this range have drastic, potentially fatal, consequences.

DESTROYERS OF HEALTH ARE EVERYWHERE

An example of how easy it is to upset your alkaline balance is illustrated here. By pouring a single 8-ounce glass of cola into 10 gallons of water slashes the water's pH from 7.4 to 4.6, a value that's considered very acidic. Can you believe that? Can you believe some people spend their lives drinking such waste?

Your body consists of about 10 gallons of water, which is supposed to be slightly alkaline. Although the body goes to every length to maintain a balance and keep its fluids at an acceptable pH, you can imagine the impossibility of the task if you drink cola. Here are the pH values for various drinks. Remember, numbers lower than 7.0 are acidic; higher numbers represent better alkalinity.

Cola	2.5
Diet soft drink	3.2
Beer	4.7
Reverse Osmosis filtered water	5.4
Distilled water	5.2
Bottled water	7.8
Ionised alkaline water	10.0

So what should you drink?

THE ULTIMATE RAW MINERAL RE-HYDRATION

A great formula for athletes is the all-powerful green juice made from kale, celery, and cucumber. Kale provides the heavy 'muscle nourishing' minerals and has high alkaline properties that neutralise lactic acid build up. Cucumber provides excellent fluids and soluble fibre. Celery (the favourite of the gorilla) should be eaten and/or juiced often to provide the sodium necessary to balance out the high potassium content of fruit. It's also excellent for replacing fluid losses through excessive perspiration. Other sources of sodium are raw olives, kale, dandelion, spinach, and sea vegetables (laver and dulse). Another excellent juice to consume after a heavy workout is celery/apple juice. It has the perfect sodium-potassium ratio (1:5) which helps prevent and relieve muscle cramping and fatigue. Sodium is a vital mineral that needs replacing if you exercise often as it can be lost heavily through sweat. After I've been to the gym I often juice two apples and half a head of celery, then pour the juice in a blender with 300grams of greens, an avocado, and maybe a chilli pepper or two. Now that's a powerful potion! Wheatgrass juice and E3Live are also excellent foods for athletes as they are rich in vital nutrients. Use them.

ARE YOU READY FOR THE CHALLENGE?

It's up to you to use food to your advantage! High levels of insulin generated by too much carbohydrate will decrease the production of good eicosanoids and increase the production of bad ones. With the balance tipping from favourable eicosanoids to unfavourable, you won't as efficiently access body fat during exercise, and your oxygen transfer rate will be dramatically reduced. In this state exercise will feel like an up hill battle, rather than a paddle downstream! If you want results, control your insulin levels!

♦ In an effort to burn as many calories as possible, many people workout too hard, yet the calorie content of their next meal usually replaces what they've just expended through exercise! It's not calories that are important but the hormonal cascade you set in motion before and after you exercise that determines the benefits you get from your workout.

♦ The most efficient source of energy is fat. It is more plentiful, and supplies more than twice the energy of carbohydrates. When exercising, carbohydrate or fats are needed to replenish the supplies of ATP essential for muscle contraction. No ATP – No muscle contraction! Fat is most efficient at replenishing ATP.

♦ 30 – 45 minutes before you start to exercise and 15 – 30 minutes after your workout eat a very small snack designed to stimulate glucagon, eat/juice/blend a small portion of high quality organic greens/wheatgrass juice/E3Live with some raw plant fat. An excellent formula is coconut water mixed with greens. These habits will prepare your body for the maximum release of growth hormone 15 to 30 minutes after your finish your anaerobic workout.

♦ Up to 2 hours after you've exercised, eat another small meal of mineral rich greens, raw plant fats and low stimulating carbohydrates. Glycogen levels will be replenished at a faster rate than if you were to eat carbohydrate alone!

♦ A gorilla can bench-press the equivalent of 4000lbs. If a gorilla is able to synthesise proteins from raw plant foods, so can you! Think of fat as the delivery vehicle and green leafy vegetables as the mineral provider necessary for building exceptional strength. If either two are missing, strength will be compromised.

♦ A great formula for athletes is the all-powerful green juice made from kale, celery, and cucumber. Another excellent juice to devour after a heavy workout is celery/apple juice as it has the perfect sodium-potassium ratio (1:5) which helps prevent and relieve muscle cramping and fatigue.

♦ Celery (the favourite of the gorilla) should be eaten and/or juiced often to provide the necessary sodium to balance out the high potassium content of fruit.

♦ Everett Smith, director of biogerontology laboratories at the University of Wisconsin, reported in 1993 that a group of middle-aged women, who did nothing more than hoist 5-pound weights, once a week, for over four years, slowed the loss of bone mass in their arms by a staggering 50%.

♦ According to Dr Robert Schulze, a daily walk of 45 mins can cause dramatic increases in bone density. But to build bone, your bone cells also need nutrition.

♦ An 8-oz. glass of carrot juice has 100-400mg of calcium and you'll assimilate all the calcium. Add some nuts or an avocado, to slow the release of the carrots sugars (since it is a hybrid food) and you're on your way to RAW PERFECTION!

♦ Parasitic infections can cause emaciation and prevent the gaining of weight. The best way to prevent this is to have a series of colonics and include garlic, onions, hot peppers, ginger, and spicy wild greens (wild mustard is excellent) in your diet. These foods will burn out a parasitic infection.

♦ Nuts are acidic – EAT THEM IN VERY SMALL QUANTITIES. For every 10g of nuts, eat/blend/juice 100g of green leafy vegetables.

♦ Human growth hormone can be seen as 'the fountain of youth'. It is a profound tissue building (anabolic) hormone produced in the pituitary, a small gland located at the base of the skull, and secreted at intervals throughout the day. HGH stimulates tissue growth, increases muscle tone and lean mass, enhances flexibility, thickens muscles, stimulates the growth of bones and organs, mobilises fat stores, shifts the metabolism to the preferential use of fat, and helps maintain healthy tissues.

+ HGH is released into your blood 90 minutes after you go to sleep and once before you wake up in the morning. To increase the release of human growth hormone from your pituitary gland, decrease your blood glucose levels, increase your blood protein levels, restrict carbohydrates in your diet, fast from time to time, eliminate cooked fats, engage in habits that increase PGE1 (a good eicosanoid), get a good night's sleep, rest often, and finally, exercise!

+ People who eat sweet, starchy, or otherwise carbohydrate laden foods before they go to bed, inhibit the normal shot of growth hormone released an hour or so after falling asleep. The same goes for people who eat high carbohydrate foods before or immediately after a workout. The pulse of growth hormone released by exercise generally hits the circulation towards the end of the workout and immediately after. To inhibit this growth hormone surge, people only have to eat a power bar, chocolate bar or drink a fizzy soft drink.

+ By strengthening and developing your muscles, you immediately build a bigger dumping ground for blood sugar, causing your body to store less fat. Think about muscle as an enormous protective barrier against rising blood sugar levels. Intense exercise can add years to your life and life to your years.

+ People in their sixties are learning to lift weights and create the muscle mass and energy levels equivalent to that of twenty-one-year-olds.

By controlling what you eat, you can begin to enhance your workouts and your recovery rate. These distinctions separate those who achieve their fitness goals from those who never seem to get out of the blocks. Use them and you'll join the elite group of people who don't have to spend all day at the gym to produce incredible results. Good Luck!

THE RAW PERFECTION EVALUATION
Do your eating habits enhance the quality of your workouts?
Do you maximise your chances of releasing HGH?
Do you use resistance training to enhance your body?

PART THREE

UNLEASH THE POWER OF YOUR MIND AND BODY

Every cell in your body is crackling with energy. You feel you can conquer the world, and in an effort to do so, your life has become incredibly busy. BUT BEWARE! By constantly pushing yourself to the limits without taking adequate rest, you may run the risk of exposing yourself to a never-ending cycle of stress. Although stress can be useful at times, too much can cause biochemical destruction.

CHAPTER 11

REMAIN CALM AND ALERT IN A WORLD OF CHAOS: ELIMINATE STRESS

Congratulations! If you've read every chapter so far, you'll have discovered what it takes to create incredible energy levels and maintain tight control over the subtle hormonal balancing act that governs your health and vitality. But beware! Many people find that with their newfound energy and desire to achieve their dreams, comes increased stress as they burn the midnight oil and push themselves to the limit. The purpose of this chapter is show you what happens when stress hormone imbalances take hold of your body, and then guide you towards the ultimate solution.

Like the smoker who dies of lung cancer after 40 years of continual smoking, stress hormone imbalances can gradually strangle your health in much the same way. Fortunately, research has been carried out in the area of neuroscience, highlighting how easy it is to restore balance to a flagging system. That's where we're headed, but to begin with you need to discover the secrets to balancing the three adrenal hormones - cortisol, DHEA and adrenaline.

THE ULTIMATE POWER OF CORTISOL

In the animal kingdom, no journey is more dramatic than that of Pacific salmon as they overcome powerful currents, leap past dams, battle against waterfalls, and fight their way upstream to return to their birth site to spawn. But do salmon thrive after such an adventure? Certainly not. After spawning, they begin to age at an accelerated rate and usually end up dying within days. What causes this accelerated ageing? Cortisol. That's right, the hormone that allowed them to reach their birth site against all odds is now the cause of their death. Put simply, the mechanism that usually monitors cortisol production becomes exhausted, leading to a massive outpouring of the hormone. When the adrenal glands are exhausted from the overproduction, the salmon's finely tuned hormonal communication system completely breaks down.

At this point the immune system is virtually destroyed leading to incredible weakness and vulnerability to disease, whilst parasites and infections begin to invade the salmon with tremendous ferocity.

HOW MANY SALMON DO YOU KNOW?

Can you think of anyone who seems to work excessively, is always stressed and never seems to relax? You don't have to be a genius to see that they are putting their body, brain, and nervous system under tremendous strain. I suggest you take a look at your own life and ask yourself whether or not you think you experience too much stress. I hope you don't, but if you do, I'm glad I brought it to your attention. In the right amounts, cortisol helps to increase your capacity to withstand stress. It assists in the metabolism of fat, protein and carbohydrate and thus energy production. It also helps thyroid activity, muscle and joint function, the rate of bone turnover, immunity to infection, quality of sleep, and the health of your skin. If however, cortisol is over-stimulated, it can destroy you both mentally and physically.

STRESS: THE TICKING TIME BOMB

Three stages make up 'the general adaptation syndrome', a term used by Hans Selye, author of 'The Stress of Life' and leading expert in the area of stress and health. Take a look for yourself and you'll see how over-exposure to stress can eventually kill!

STAGE 1 – THE ALARM REACTION

In this stage a person secretes adrenaline, cortisol and DHEA, causing their whole physiology to react and prepare for the threat of pain, whether, physical, verbal or even mental. The body responds by increasing heart rate, breathing rate and muscle tension. Stress is perceived differently by different people, highlighting the fact that it is only the perception of threat that causes stress rather than the threat itself.

STAGE 2 – THE RESISTANCE STAGE

Prolonged stress promotes the increased release of cortisol, which in turn causes a negative immune factor, Interleukin-6 (IL-6) to be secreted.

Abnormal levels of IL-6 are associated with autoimmune conditions, inflammatory diseases and allergies. IL-6 also causes calcium to be pulled from the bones, increasing the chances of osteoporosis. Remember this because I'll come back to IL-6 later.

DHEA is a precursor of the stress hormones adrenaline and cortisol. Every time the body makes these hormones, DHEA levels are depleted. When cortisol and IL-6 levels rise, DHEA production dwindles to almost nothing. The real problems begin when the natural cortisol shut off mechanism becomes disrupted, damaging a part of the brain called the hippocampus.

Let me explain. Usually when the threat/stressor has vanished, the hippocampus tells the system to stop producing cortisol, but in cases of extreme stress, excess cortisol damages the hippocampus and it fails to register the elevated levels. The damage turns what is supposed to be a feedback mechanism into a feedforward mechanism. Rather than shutting down cortisol production the brain allows it to continue, even in the absence of any threat. As your body adapts to the stress your brain structure begins to alter until finally, hormonal imbalances become the norm.

Overexposure to stress also inhibits the enzyme delta 6 desaturase and knocks out the production of good eicosanoids, predisposing its victim to many illnesses including depression, ulcers, premature ageing, cancer, heart disease, skin diseases, Alzheimer's disease, hypertension, diabetes, multiple sclerosis and Parkinson's disease.

You'd think by removing the stimulus, stress hormones would decline and return to normal, but at the end of this second stage the threat could have vanished and a person can still have high levels of the stress hormones in their bloodstream. Have you ever seen anyone go on holiday and find it hard to relax because they are so used to being busy? Stress hormones make you pursue activities rather than rest.

STAGE 3 –THE PHASE OF EXHAUSTION

This is the most evil stage of all. The chosen organs that continue to fight the battle against the stressor gradually weaken. As they wear out, the body turns to other organs. This drafting in of other organs causes another surge of adrenaline and cortisol secretion. Eventually not enough stress hormones are produced and low levels are detected in the blood. The adrenal glands enlarge, the thymus, spleen, and lymph nodes shrink, and the number of white blood cells diminish in number resulting in chronic fatigue and susceptibility to infections, as the immune system is weakened. Even excess stomach acid is secreted as blood pressure rises and sex hormones decline. Hardly an advert for RAW PERFECTION is it! I hope what you're reading is motivating you to take control. The place to begin is by increasing the production of...

THE ANTI-AGEING HORMONE: DHEA

In the late 1980s Arthur Schwartz, a biochemist at Temple University, administered DHEA to mice. He observed a remarkable reversal of ageing: Old mice regained their sleek, glossy coats and youthful vigour, cancers disappeared (whether naturally occurring or induced by artificial means), obese mice returned to normal weight, diabetes improved, and immunity to disease increased.

Under normal circumstances, between 10 and 20mg of cortisol is produced by the body on a daily basis. DHEA production ranges from between 25 to 30mg, making it the most abundant steroid in your body. Both are produced at different levels during the day and it's the rhythm between the two that is critical. Cortisol is usually higher in the morning and lower at night. If any one factor disturbs this synchronicity, health can be compromised. Too much stress and not enough relaxation/recuperation eventually upsets the fine hormonal balancing act, causing an increase in cortisol output. Think of excess cortisol production as the first step to dropping your 'immunity' guard, inviting the one-two punch of infection and disease.

DHEA is critical! It prevents cortisol from causing widespread damage by binding to its receptor sites, ultimately protecting part of the eicosanoid production pathway by preventing cortisol from inhibiting delta 6 desaturase. As you'll remember, delta 6 desaturase is the enzyme that allows linoleic acid to flow freely into the eicosanoid production pipeline. DHEA indirectly keeps delta 6 desaturase active. Without it you'd have no mechanism to prevent the devastating effect of excess cortisol on eicosanoid production.

ARE YOU BEGINNING TO SEE
HOW ALL THIS FITS TOGETHER?

1. Excess Insulin production = increase in cortisol output
2. Excess stress = increase in cortisol production

When cortisol levels increase, DHEA binds to cortisol receptor sites protecting part of the eicosanoid production pathway. If this continues, the ratio of cortisol to DHEA increases – eicosanoid balance suffers – insulin rises even more – and health gradually spirals downwards. At this point the hormonal philharmonic isn't sounding too terribly good and accelerated ageing is too often the result!

A decrease in DHEA, with a corresponding increase in cortisol can cause biochemical destruction. Let this destruction happen to someone else, not you! It's your responsibility to maintain optimal DHEA levels by:

1. Preventing the secretion of excess insulin! Excess insulin interferes with an enzyme that helps produce DHEA. Experiments with rhesus monkeys who were put on calorie-restricted diets caused DHEA levels to rise, whilst simultaneously lowering insulin levels. (See Chapter 15 – Maximise Your Lifespan)
2. Take 200mcg of chromium daily! Studies have shown that patients' levels of DHEA drop by an average of 10% after they discontinue to take the supplement. Eat foods such as pulses, nuts, seeds and asparagus to keep your chromium levels topped up.

STIMULATE DHEA AND BOOST YOUR IMMUNE SYSTEM

DHEA, controls age-related disorders, helps repair and maintain tissues, reduces arteriosclerosis, increases insulin sensitivity, controls allergic reaction, and most importantly, balances the immune system. Low levels of DHEA cause sexual dysfunction, muscle shrinkage, memory loss, degenerative diseases and poor immune function. Research has found DHEA to help reduce obesity, ageing, and cancer (particularly breast cancer).

TRACKING THE DECLINE OF DHEA

DHEA production is naturally high (regardless of diet) until about age 30, highlighting why young people are less prone to disease. At age 30 in many people (not all) there is a decline in production. In fact, no other age-related hormone declines as fast as DHEA, with the average drop being from about 30mg per day at age twenty to less than 6mg per day at age eighty. It isn't unusual for sufferers of cancer, heart disease, atherosclerosis and Alzheimers to all have low levels of DHEA in their blood. Stimulate DHEA and you also trigger the release of human growth hormone (HGH), the true elixir of youth!

A twelve-year study looking at hundreds of ageing humans highlights the importance of maintaining adequate blood/DHEA levels. When DHEA levels dropped, mortality increased. According to Dr. William Regelson of the Medical Collage of Virginia, DHEA is "one of the best biochemical biomarkers for chronological age."

REMEMBER TO BOOST DHEA
AND YOU'LL FIND IT EASIER TO REMEMBER!

In an experiment with brain cell tissue cultures, anti-ageing researcher Dr. Eugene Roberts discovered that even very low concentrations of DHEA will "increase the number of neurons in the brain, improve their ability to establish connections and their differentiation." He concludes that DHEA plays "a significant role in normal function of neuronal cells". By actively keeping your DHEA levels adequate/high, evidence suggests that your ability to learn and remember will increase and you'll enhance every aspect of your mental performance.

ENHANCE YOUR BRAIN POWER FURTHER
AND CEMENT YOUR MEMORIES

Chronic stress also depletes the stimulating neurotransmitter norepinephrine (see chapter 14 – Food For Thought). Take a look at how a simple neurotransmitter imbalance can sabotage your mental health:

◆ As norepinephrine is depleted, a deficit is created in the frontal lobe of the neocortex, where much abstract thinking takes place.

◆ Norepinephrine is used to cement memories, without it your ability to remember declines. Students with chronic stress scored 13% lower on IQ tests than students with low stress in one revealing study. Excess cortisol causes learning ability and concentration to hit rock bottom!

◆ Norepinephrine plays a critical role in keeping you happy and in good spirits. Chronic stress causes norepinephrine to be shunted away from your limbic system (part of your brain that controls your emotions). With a lack of norepinephrine in the emotional centre of your brain, people often experience a biological depression leading to feelings of anxiety and malaise.

DO YOU WANT TO MAXIMISE YOUR PLEASURE
PATHWAYS OR DISRUPT THEM?

If brain chemistry is disrupted for too long a period, the disruption can lead to a condition known as anhedonia, the inability to feel pleasure. Anhedonia leaves its victim biochemically unable of being excited, joyous or happy and is very common among chronic abusers of stimulating drugs such as cocaine.

Simply imagine that the drug abuser has supplied so much artificial stimulation to their brain via the drug, that their brain has forgotten how to produce its own pleasure chemicals such as norepinephrine and other stimulating catecholamine neurotransmitters. Norepinephrine is a critical ingredient in the pursuit of unlimited happiness.

HAVE YOU EVER FELT NUMB AFTER COMPLETING A LONG STRETCH OF WORK?

Many people experience a mild form of anhedonia after completing a long, stressful piece of work. When they finally finish, they know they should feel ecstatic, but end up feeling numb. Their brain's happiness chemicals were burned up by excessive stress.

The great advantage of training in N.L.P. or hypnosis is that you can begin to train yourself to experience more pleasure and joy on a day to day basis for absolutely no reason. People think this is crazy, but it's not as crazy as getting stressed for no reason – and there are millions of people doing that every minute of every day. The more pleasure you experience on a day to day basis, the less you will physically react to stress. The less you react to stress, the less you will damage your brain with cortisol!

IF YOUR BRAIN ISN'T HAPPY, YOU WON'T BE HAPPY!
THREE POINTS WHERE STRESS CAN DESTROY YOUR BRAIN

There are essentially three ways that stress can destroy optimal function of the brain.

◆ Stress disrupts the supply of the brain's only source of fuel, glucose

Firstly, your ability to adapt and deal with the unpredictable nature of life will determine whether you perceive situations as stressful or not. If your find yourself relaxed and in total control, then congratulations. But if you've been stressed at times when a more relaxed state of mind was appropriate, you are risking the integrity of your brainpower!

Stress causes cortisol to be released from the adrenals, inhibiting the uptake of blood sugar from part of your brain called the hippocampus. The hippocampus happens to be the brain's primary memory centre and without enough blood sugar it suffers an energy shortage. This energy shortage means the brain has no way to chemically lay down a memory, leading directly to short and long term memory problems.

The importance of conditioning relaxed states of mind cannot be overemphasised, especially if you want to learn something like a new language or a new skill. Another unwanted mental effect of chronic stress is its influence on brain waves. A person experiencing stress has a predominance of "uptight" beta waves, rather than 'calm' alpha and theta waves. (See chapter 12 – The Electrifying Power of Mind Technology for more information on brainwaves and peak performance brain states)

♦ **Stress interferes with the function of neurotransmitters**
Imagine what happens in a freak snowstorm when all the power cables are down. The telephone, television or computer won't work and the weather is too bad to travel. It's at this point you have a complete communication breakdown. This is the kind of effect stress and cortisol has on the mind. It prevents neurotransmitters from sending information between various areas of the brain, causing problems with concentration and focus. Can you see why people are often so muddled and confused in stressful situations?

Have you ever wondered why hypnosis is used for memory retrieval? Quite simply, a skilled hypnotist can access a relaxed/lucid state of consciousness, increasing the chances of memory retrieval.

One of the reasons we need sleep is to rebalance brain chemistry and re-establish neurotransmitter equilibrium. If you can actively learn to maintain optimal neurotransmitter equilibrium you'll maintain a magical mind and powerful brain for the rest of your life. You'll learn more about neurotransmitter equilibrium in chapters 12 and 14.

♦ **Stress causes the eventual death of neurons, by creating free-radical molecules**
Cortisol allows excessive amounts of calcium to enter the brain cells, increasing free radical formation. Excess free radical formation can lead to brain cell death. Antioxidants protect you from aggressive free-radical attack, highlighting the importance of a raw food diet.

Half the dry weight of your brain is fat and a third of that is made from polyunsaturated essential fatty acids making it incredibly vulnerable to free radical attack. Eicosanoids are made from polyunsaturated fatty acids and since they're easy targets for free radicals, it's up to you to protect them with antioxidants.

I FOUND MY FREEDOM ON BLUEBERRY HILL

Scientists have found that the antioxidants within blueberries can actually reverse the effects of the passing years and help retain optimal health. For example, rodents begin to lose their balance and co-ordination at 12 months and according to researchers, by 19 months (human equivalent – 65 to 75 years old) the time they can balance on a narrow rod falls from 13 seconds to 5 seconds. However, when the researchers gave the rodents daily doses of blueberry extract for eight weeks (equivalent to half a cup of berries for humans) their times dramatically improved, returning to an average of 11 seconds. Their ability to find their way around a maze, a test of short-term memory, also improved.

Imagine that! By including a daily cup full of the berries into your diet you could benefit from improved balance, improved co-ordination and a more powerful short-term memory! The place to begin is by…

ELIMINATING QUICK FIX REFINED 'EMPTY CALORIE' FOODS

Is it a habit of yours to reach for a chocolate bar or cup of coffee in order to raise your energy level and mood? Stop! This habit could be killing you! Whilst providing the artificial stimulation, the high sugar content/caffeine level causes blood-sugar abnormalities, the unnaturally high release of insulin, followed by the stress hormone cortisol to restore blood sugar levels. Combine a diet loaded with sugar, caffeine and other stimulants with high levels of stress and you've got a killing formula. Sugar eats up nutrients that are otherwise needed for you body to operate at its best.

STRESS EATS AWAY AT STORED VITAL NUTRIENTS

Stress places the same demands on your body as exercise. It magnifies your nutritional needs and burns up extra nutrients very rapidly. Whether you think you suffer from stress or not, you need to benefit from spells of relaxation.

When cortisol is released in response to stress, it causes the mineral magnesium to be excreted in excessive amounts. The irony is that magnesium happens to be a calming mineral and low levels increase your vulnerability to stress. This is how the downward spiral continues, stress causes magnesium loss – magnesium loss increases your chances of perceiving situations as more stressful – cortisol is released and magnesium is excreted.

A fascinating study by the U.S. Department of Agriculture shed more light on this phenomenon. Researchers created a scenario where subjects were given more work than usual, with very strict deadlines. When they completed the work, blood samples showed a 33% drop in mineral content.

By eating E3Live you supply a powerful shot of chlorophyll to your body to help eliminate toxic minerals, whilst replacing them with the vital nutrients your body needs to remain strong in the throws of adversity.

INCREASE YOUR CONSUMPTION OF RAW PLANT FATS

Controlling the release of cortisol and the decline of DHEA can be assisted by using plant sterols and sterolins (raw plant fats), according to Professor Patrick Bouic, co-author of The Immune System Cure. He performed research using plant sterols and sterolins and found that these powerful plant nutrients not only control cortisol but also decrease the negative immune factor IL-6.

♦ Did you know that the HIV virus uses IL-6 to replicate itself?
♦ Did you know that the AFA algae found in E3Live, has been shown to inhibit the growth of the AIDS virus according to research findings published in The Journal of the National Cancer Institute in 1989?
♦ Can you make the link?

Sterols and sterolins are used to produce DHEA and by eating a diet high in sterols and sterolins, your DHEA levels can become optimal within as little as 4-6 weeks. Some of the best sources or plant sterols and sterolins are sesame seeds, sunflower seeds, almonds, pomegranates, figs, grapefruit, oranges, apricots, bananas, apples, white squash, olives, soybean sprouts, radish greens, clove, ginger, oregano and thyme.

HAVE YOU EVER CRAVED CARBOHYDRATES DURING STRESSFUL TIMES?

The high levels of cortisol that are released during stress also cause people to crave carbohydrates. Cortisol is responsible for triggering the release of the brain chemical neuropeptide Y. When this happens, people's desire to eat carbohydrate food increases, explaining why many people overeat sweets and starchy foods at times of high stress.

CONTROL NEUROPEPTIDE Y AND STOP ANY CRAVINGS

Stress may cause the release of neuropeptide Y, but so do unbalanced meals. If you get hungry within 4-6 hours of your last meal, it'll be up to you to assess what happened. Take a look at the chain of events that can cause many of the problems over-eating.

♦ High carbohydrate meal – Too much insulin produced – blood sugar levels driven down – mental alertness declines – drowsiness sets in – you're making too many bad eicosanoids and you crave sugary foods.

♦ Very low carbohydrate meal – Too little insulin – you make too many good eicosanoids – not enough insulin crosses the blood-brain barrier to interact with the hypothalamus – the synthesis of neuropeptide Y increases – appetite is stimulated.

Neuropeptide Y is such a powerful stimulator of appetite, it won't matter that your mental acuity is excellent and that your brain is getting enough glucose, your desire for food will still increase.

In most people, the hormone leptin shuts off neuropeptide Y production. Leptin is a hormone secreted from fat that stimulates the hypothalamus, thereby controlling appetite. Scientists have observed that as more leptin is produced, appetite decreases. Unfortunately, in some obese people, it doesn't matter how much of the hormone they produce, neuropeptide Y production continues. These unfortunate few feel ravenously hungry all of the time, causing them to massively overeat, a condition known as hyperphagia. It's up to you to engineer meals that keep you satisfied for the next 4-6 hours.

USE MEALS STRATEGICALLY TO ELIMINATE STRESS

Re-balancing cortisol and DHEA is easy if you are willing to apply two simple principles that allow you to get immediate control over your blood sugar levels:

1. GRAZE RATHER THAN GORGE

Ensure you keep your blood sugar levels balanced by eating small meals regularly throughout the day. Grazing prevents excessive insulin output, which indirectly prevents cortisol from being released to restore blood sugar levels. By controlling cortisol output you indirectly fine-tune your overall hormonal philharmonic. A life of excessive cortisol secretion could physically degenerate your brain, eventually causing it to lose its ability to orchestrate the hormone-secreting endocrine glands. These are the primary communication links between all parts of your body. Nobody wants a decline in energy, mood, sex drive, and immune function, but that's the result if you don't control cortisol. And before you argue that the decline of these functions is simply part of growing old, think again! There are many people living healthfully and sexually-active well into their hundreds!

2. EAT MEALS THAT HAVE A 2:1 CARBOHYDRATE:PROTEIN RATIO

Recent research has found that eating some protein with carbohydrate provides additional adrenal support by reducing the stimulation of cortisol. If your are stressed eat some fruit and nuts for example. Sprouted nuts, seeds, beans and lentils contain both protein and carbohydrate. They are great anti-stress foods. Many foods contain quality protein as well as carbohydrate, such as sprouted seeds, peas, beans as well as broccoli. Take this advice to heart because nourishing your adrenal glands is vital if you want to live a busy fun-packed lifestyle.

THE POWER OF TRANSCENDENTAL MEDITATION

Before I whisk you away on a wonderful journey into the world of neuroscience and brain technology, I want you to take a look at the power of meditation – specifically Transcendental Meditation (TM). More than 500 studies and research projects have highlighted the incredible power of this discipline. Here are just a few:

♦ TM consistently produces a significant lowering of blood pressure – typically around 10mm Hg for systolic blood. This could have a major significance for the health of the world, as hypertension is the main risk factor for stroke and a major factor in coronary heart disease.

♦ TM has been shown to produce positive health, including increased creativity and intelligence, more satisfaction from relationships, a feeling of mental and physical rejuvenation and a dramatically increased ability to manage depression, insomnia, migraines and irritable bowel.

♦ The act of meditating allows you to slow your metabolism down to the point where you reach a hypometabolic state. The only other time this state is reached is during sleep or hibernation. When you enter the hypometabolic state your consumption of oxygen decreases rapidly. To be more precise, sleep causes an 8% drop in oxygen consumption, but meditation can cause a decrease of between 10% and 20%, highlighting the deeply relaxed state that it creates. In this state your entire physical system is rejuvenated.

♦ Meditation influences your body on many different levels. To begin with it causes a decrease in blood lactate. Lactate is secreted by muscles and can cause mild anxiety. Researchers demonstrated the power of lactate in an interesting study with a group of patients, all suffering anxiety disorders. The group was split in two. One half received a placebo injection, the other group received an injection with lactate. As you can imagine, the first group had no response, but the second group quickly experienced an anxiety attack. As you meditate, you can expect blood lactate levels to drop significantly within as little as ten minutes.

♦ The sleep hormone melatonin is increased by meditation. Studies at the University of Massachusetts Medical Centre have shown that meditators produce significantly more melatonin than non-meditators on a regular basis, offering people exceptional relief from insomnia.

♦ One of the main benefits of meditation is that it causes a decline in cortisol production, which will stay with you long after your meditation session ends. If you meditate on a regular basis you can expect cortisol levels to remain low, day after day, week after week. This is another reason why meditation significantly slows the ageing process, increasing lifespan and health span.

♦ A study of 2000 people practising Transcendental Meditation showed that they had fewer than half the number of doctor visits and days in hospital than a control group. They needed less medical and surgical treatment in all 17-disease categories, including 87% fewer hospitalisations for cardio-vascular disease, 55% fewer for tumours,

73% fewer nose, throat and lung problems and fewer disorders of the nervous system.

♦ Meditation is known to decrease ageing. You only have to look at the DHEA levels of meditators compared to those of non-meditators. When you're 20 years old, your DHEA level is about 800. When you're 40, it's about 300. And when you're 70, it's about 2. People who practice TM regularly have been shown to have much higher levels of DHEA than average people of the same age. Levels of DHEA normally decrease with age and high levels are directly linked to a low risk of heart disease, cardiovascular disease, osteoporosis, and breast cancer.

♦ Because DHEA is an adrenal steroidal hormone, it is part of the body's response mechanism to stress. Generally, stress (excess cortisol production) depletes DHEA. In fact, many clinicians monitor DHEA levels as a measure of long term stress. If DHEA levels are low, it can indicate that the patient suffered long-term, chronic stress. If you can keep cortisol secretion to a minimum, using meditation and other techniques that induce the 'relaxation response' you automatically protect DHEA. Another study of meditators showed that men over the age of 45 had on average 23% more DHEA than non-meditators, whilst women had a staggering 47% more!

♦ In one study, 242 men aged 50 to 79 were monitored for their DHEA Levels. Afterward their health was tracked for twelve years. Those with the highest levels of DHEA had the best long-term health, even if they smoked and had high cholesterol. For every 20% increase in DHEA levels in these men, there was a 48% decrease in heart disease, and a 36% decrease in death from any cause.

♦ Alzheimer's patients, however, invariably have much lower levels of DHEA than do non-Alzheimer's patients of the same age. One study indicated that Alzheimer's patients had 48% less DHEA than a matched control group.

♦ People who meditate and increase DHEA levels report renewed energy and sex drive, an increased sense of well-being, an elevated mood, and a greater ability to cope with stress. More importantly, DHEA has been shown to have immune-boosting properties. Research had shown, for example, that DHEA restores the cancer-fighting T cells and enhances the activity of the natural killer cells (NK cells).

♦ DHEA can reverse osteoporosis by increasing the activity of bone-building cells (osteoblasts), whilst inhibiting the activity of bone-destroying cells (osteoclasts). Although cortisol is only one of the many

> hormones secreted by the adrenal glands, it's secreted in response to stress. Like all hormones, moderate amounts prove to be anything but harmful, but when produced in excess, many problems can occur.

Amazing isn't it? But what's more amazing is that the marvellous effects of brain technology such as light/sound stimulation devices, the Alpha Stim and The End® Personal Growth Through Technology Programme can produce good, if not better results than transcendental meditation (TM) and in less time! It's worth knowing how powerful meditation is before you learn about the power of mind machines. The point is simple: Whether you choose to buy a mind machine or meditate, ensure you take time out every day to quiet the mind and go inside, allowing your whole body to relax and rejuvenate.

SOMETHING ELSE TO CONSIDER:
THE STRESS OF LONELINESS

Did you know that if an older person loses their spouse, they are ten times more likely to die within a year than if their spouse were to remain alive? Did you also know that when a person gets divorced, their chance of becoming ill over the course of the next year rises dramatically by 1200%? Those who are chronically stressed have higher chances of mortality and illness. This information may not inspire some people, but at least it highlights the importance of taking responsibility and doing everything in your power to maintain health and wellness. In this case start appreciating your partner and/or circle of friends/pets, they are as important to your health as your next meal!

ARE YOU READY FOR THE CHALLENGE?

Although cortisol is only one of the many hormones secreted by the adrenal glands, it's secreted in response to stress. Like all hormones, moderate amounts prove to be anything but harmful, but when produced in excess, many problems can occur. Cortisol does have a positive role in your body, but like insulin, too much can lead you down a road you'd rather not travel. The importance of doing all you can to prevent stress from compromising your immune system is obvious when you're aware of the insulin-cortisol-IL-6-DHEA connection. It's up to you to safeguard yourself against stress by ensuring your body is abundant in all the vital nutrients that build and support life. Use the principles in these pages, enhance your own production of DHEA, and eliminate any habits that cause its production to dwindle. Set aside time in the day to relax, allowing your brain to recuperate. Continue to take responsibility. You've built a powerful foundation. Now is the time to excel yourself. Here's a re-cap:

♦ Cortisol can be incredibly toxic. If your brain is exposed to excessive levels of it, brain degeneration is usually the result. In fact, overexposure to cortisol is possibly the number one cause of brain degeneration.

♦ When cortisol is released in response to stress, it causes magnesium to be excreted in excessive amounts. Magnesium is a calming mineral and low levels increase your vulnerability to stress.

♦ A fascinating study by the U.S. Department of Agriculture showed that when subjects were given more work than usual, with very strict deadlines, blood samples showed a 33% drop in mineral content.

♦ Cortisol is responsible for triggering the release of the brain chemical neuropeptide Y, which leads to carbohydrate cravings.

♦ High carbohydrate diets that stimulate too much insulin cause a rapid drop in blood-sugar levels resulting in poor brain function and cause the secretion of cortisol to increase blood sugar levels. Excess insulin also interferes with the enzyme that helps produce DHEA.

♦ DHEA prevents cortisol from causing widespread damage by binding to its receptor sites. It helps protect part of the eicosanoid production pathway by indirectly keeping delta 6 desaturase active. Without DHEA you'd have no mechanism to prevent the devastating effect of excess cortisol on eicosanoid production. The less stress you experience the more harmonious your eicosanoid status.

♦ DHEA acts as a buffer against stress related hormones (such as cortisol). If you don't actively do as much as you can to increase/maintain optimal levels of DHEA, as you age you'll make less, making you more susceptible to stress and disease.

♦ Graze rather than gorge! Grazing prevents excessive insulin output, which indirectly prevents cortisol from being released to restore blood sugar levels. Recent research has found that eating some protein with carbohydrate provides additional adrenal support by reducing the stimulation of cortisol. Calorie restricted diets also cause DHEA to rise (as long as the diet isn't nutrient deficient).

♦ Dr. Eugene Roberts discovered that by actively keeping your DHEA levels high, evidence suggests you'll boost your ability to learn and remember, whilst enhancing mental performance.

♦ It isn't unusual for sufferers of cancer, heart disease, atherosclerosis and Alzheimers to have low levels of DHEA in their blood.

♦ Stimulate DHEA and you also trigger the release of growth hormone, the true elixir of youth!

♦ Dr. William Regelson of the Medical Collage of Virginia, states that DHEA is "one of the best bio-chemical biomarkers for chronological age." When DHEA levels drop, mortality increases!

♦ DHEA helps control stress, maintain optimal mineral balance, control the production of sex hormones, build lean body mass and burn fat by enhancing energy metabolism. You'll burn calories more easily as your energy levels rise.

♦ When you decrease cortisol production, testosterone levels increase. Testosterone is responsible for many health advantages including sex drive. High insulin levels retard testosterone production, because one of the steroid precursors (pregnenolone) required for testosterone production is diverted toward increased cortisol production.

♦ Laughing and smiling diffuse stress. Research has shown that people who laugh easily respond better to treatment for disease. Laughter prompts positive physiological changes that benefit the immune system.

Master this chapter and soon you'll be looking in the mirror at someone who is not only slim, with clear beautiful skin and toned muscles, but who has an incredibly calm and powerful mind. The choice is yours, a lack of control and a stressful life, or total control and complete abundance.

THE RAW PERFECTION EVALUATION:
Is your diet full of stress relieving/brain enhancing raw foods?
Do you control insulin and glucagon, optimising blood sugar levels and minimising cortisol output?
Do you understand the importance of grazing rather than gorging?
Do you take time to meditate or relax during the day?

CHAPTER 12

THE ELECTRIFYING POWER OF MIND TECHNOLOGY

As the young author sits busily writing his first best seller, his computer workstation is surrounded by many books. The subjects vary from hypnosis, nutrition and mind enhancing technologies to meditation and the mind/body connection. He's been working constantly for 40 minutes and feels he'd be more productive if he took a short break. He lies on his bed, grabs his Alpha Stim device, wets the electrodes, and attaches them to his ear lobes. Next he grabs his Mindlab and puts on the headphones and liteframe goggles (heavy-duty sunglasses with built in LEDs that flash at various frequencies, entraining brain wave frequency).

PREPARE FOR THE JOURNEY OF A LIFETIME – DAILY!

By pressing the 'on' button, the Alpha Stim starts to induce a kind of tingling in his ears, whilst stimulating his brain with electrical impulses. He then presses a button on the console of the Mindlab to engage a program of light and sound pulses.

For the next 20 minutes the hypnotic, pulsating tones capture his attention, whilst the rich variety of colours from the flashing lights of the goggles, move and swirl in front of his eyes. As he becomes totally engaged in the delights of the audio-visual experience provided by the Mindlab, the Alpha Stim sends micro-electrical current between his two ear lobes, stimulating various areas of his brain. He is spellbound and absorbed by the experience.

This may sound like something out of a science fiction movie, but elite athletes, sports professionals, business executives and people such as you and I are using mind machines more and more frequently to combat stress and enhance peak performance – with exciting results!

MIND TECHNOLOGY HAS THE POWER TO REVOLUTIONISE YOUR MENTAL HEALTH

When the 20 minutes are over, the Alpha Stim stops, the lights of the Mindlab fade, and the sound pulses gradually diminish to nothing. Silence. He can't believe that a mere 20 minutes ago he was feeling tired and overloaded by the task at hand. He now feels relaxed and alert, energised but calm. His brain is functioning far more effectively than it was before. The kinds of changes that have taken place at a neurological level are remarkable. Take a look for yourself.

♦ **In the 20 minutes that passed, he exercised his brain making it healthier and more powerful.**

A wealth of brain research is proving that your brain, like your body, requires stimulation and challenge to function optimally. Just as your muscles grow stronger from physical exercise, by exposing your brain to stimulation that manipulates your brain waves, you exercise your brain and strengthen it.

Dr Marian Diamond, neuroanatomist and leader in the research of the physical effects of thinking on the brain, has proved that the more you think and challenge your intellect the bigger your brain becomes, and the better it functions.

Evidence suggests that mind machines can provide the kind of stimulation, challenge, and novelty that can strengthen your brain, increase the size and health of its neurons, produce peak performance states of mind, increase intelligence, and enhance well-being, regardless of your age.

Under the right conditions neurons can regenerate, suggesting that given the right type of stimulation your brain will continuously heal itself and replace lost cells, in much the same way as your skin can heal itself after it is cut.

One neuroscientist at the University of California at Los Angeles took specimens from over twenty human brains and analysed them under a microscope. He found a clear and definite relationship between the number of years of education and dendritic length. The more people had learned, the greater their dendritic length. Intellectual challenge has a direct physical effect on dendritic systems. With proper nutrition, your brain can create new dendrites, and forge new synaptic connections – indefinitely.

It doesn't matter whether you are young or old, your brain has the capacity to grow, and you have the capacity to become more intelligent. The more you learn, the greater your capacity for further learning. The more you put into your brain, the more open it becomes. But without sufficient stimulation, whatever your age, this capacity for growth will be limited.

The simple challenge presented by computer video games has proved to be enough to significantly improve the mental ability of the elderly. Mind machines can stimulate changes in brain wave frequency and access states of mind that are synonymous with accelerated learning.

♦ In the 20 minutes that passed his memory has increased.

Mind machines have been proven to improve both long-term and short-term memory. The Alpha Stim works by stimulating protein synthesis. For memories to become permanent in your brain, there has to be a process of nerve cell growth (protein synthesis) involving RNA (Ribonucleic acid). There is a greater concentration of RNA in your brain than anywhere else in your body. RNA synthesis is absolutely essential for the creation of memory and may even be a memory storage molecule itself. It declines naturally with age or illness and represents one of the reasons why older people have problems storing memories. RNA is such a powerful antioxidant and key to longevity that experiments with rats have shown it can increase life span by 20%.

AFA algae (E3Live) contains 4% RNA/DNA (nucleic acids). These are needed by the body to make new cells, repair damaged cells and for growth of body tissue. Without enough RNA/DNA, you may suffer the consequences of a weak immune system and ultimately age prematurely. Poor nutrition, pollution and stress can deplete your RNA/DNA. Ensure you use E3Live daily.

♦ After the 20 minutes of stimulation he has a higher IQ.

In several studies, subjects with learning disabilities have increased their IQ between 20 and 30 points with the use of mind machines. Other research suggests that mind machines can also dramatically boost the IQ of normal, healthy users.

♦ His intelligence, creativity and problem solving ability has expanded after 20 minutes.

Scores on several psychological tests measuring creativity show significant boosts when subjects used mind technology before the tests. If you stimulate different brainwave states with external stimulation, you may facilitate your ability to allow more variations in brain functioning by breaking up patterns of information flow at the neurological level. This can help you develop the ability to move rapidly from one state of mind to the other through increased neural flexibility. In fact, one of the useful by products of learning N.L.P. and hypnosis is developing the ability to create and alter your state of consciousness rapidly, allowing you to adapt more easily in any situation.

DISCOVERING THE MYRIAD OF MENTAL STATES WITH MIND MACHINES

Every imaginable mental state you experience is the result of a specific pattern of electrical and chemical activity in your brain. Brain activity can be altered and shaped by external stimuli, including sounds, lights, electromagnetic fields, and physical movements. Mind machines can direct these stimuli to appropriate areas in your brain and reliably trigger specific brain states. When you use these technologies it's possible to guide yourself into such brain states as euphoria, reverie, recall of long-past experiences, stimulation of memories, sexual excitement, deep concentration, and heightened creativity – the list is endless. Studies by neurologists have now proved that in certain extraordinary mental states, such as deep meditation or intense creativity, both hemispheres begin to produce strong brain waves in a single, coherent rhythm, operating in unison. Scientists call this state of whole brain thinking synchrony, and it has recently become clear that certain brain stimulation devices can rapidly boost your brain into this beneficial state.

♦ **His brain's processing speed has increased after 20 minutes.**

In a variety of settings, subjects using mind technology have learned more, learned faster, and proven more adept at learning difficult and complex material than ordinary subjects. Accelerated learning is encouraged since brain cells can forge new, richer interconnections. Under the proper conditions, you can absorb, store, process, and recall vast amounts of information, given the right stimulation.

♦ **His body is now profoundly relaxed and the levels of adrenaline and other stress related substances in his body have decreased after 20 minutes.**

Evidence shows that various mind machines can dramatically reduce levels of stress-related neurochemicals, reduce muscle tension, lower high blood pressure, slow heart rate, soothe jangled nerves, and quickly produce whole body levels of relaxation whilst increasing resistance to stress. This helps with the production of good eicosanoids. Remember, the delta 6-desaturase enzyme isn't inhibited along the eicosanoid production pathway when stress chemicals are minimised in the body.

♦ **His immune system is functioning more effectively after a mere 20 minutes.**

Researchers are exploring the effects of mind machines on individual components of the immune system with healthy and sick subjects (including those with AIDS, chronic fatigue immune dysfunction syndrome, and cancer). They have found clear evidence that these devices can increase the power of the immune system to overcome existing diseases and boost its resistance to infection.

By reducing cortisol, your ability to produce favourable eicosanoids remains efficient, leading to a powerful immune system response!

CAN YOU BELIEVE THAT A MERE 20 MINUTES CAN MAKE SOMEONE INSTANTLY SMARTER AND HEALTHIER?

The story of this 20 minute break is the story of what it took for me to write this book. I frequently took these power breaks to boost my brain capacity, enter peak performance states of mind and condition relaxed, focused states of awareness. You may develop amazing energy levels by following the principles of RAW PERFECTION, but make sure you set aside time to relax and recuperate.

BEGINNING TO SURF THE BRAIN WAVES

Beta Waves – In the waking state your brain is alert and busy. Beta waves are the most dominant and range from about 14 cycles per second (14Hz) to more than 100 Hz. Beta waves are associated with alertness, arousal, concentration, cognition, and in excess – anxiety.

Alpha Waves – As you relax, brain-wave activity slows down and you produce bursts of alpha waves. Alpha waves range in frequency from approximately 8 – 13 Hz. When your mind is unfocused and you're day dreaming or taking a break, alpha waves become dominant throughout your brain, producing a calm and pleasant sensation. Alpha activity can usually be found in those who are healthy and not under a great deal of stress. The lack of significant alpha activity can be a sign of anxiety, stress, brain damage or illness.

Theta Waves – The more relaxed you become, the deeper your state of drowsiness and the quicker your brain shifts to slower, more powerfully rhythmic theta waves. These waves range in frequency from about 4 – 8 Hz. They reflect the meditative state, which lies between wakefulness and sleep. Often, when people experience theta waves, they can access information otherwise out of their consciousness (unconscious retrieval). Hypnosis is very powerful and excellent for training its subjects to access theta brain activity. As you train your brain to access a theta state, you'll begin to experience deep personal insights, increased creativity and increased creative problem solving. Theta brain waves combine a pleasant, relaxed feeling with extreme alertness.

ZEN MONKS SPEND 20 YEARS IN ORDER TO MASTER THETA CONTROL – YOU CAN DO IT IN TEN MINUTES!

A series of EEG studies by Japanese scientists showed that the most skilled Zen monks sank right through alpha and began producing the slower theta waves when they went into deep meditative states. Even in the depths of theta where most people simply relax further and fall asleep, monks however, are extremely alert.

The more meditative experience monks had, the more theta they generated. If they had accumulated 20 years of meditative experience, they were able to access deep theta quickly. 20 years is a lot of training, but fortunately, through scientific breakthroughs in the field of neuroscience, scientists discovered it did not require years of training or any special meditative powers to produce such unique patterns of brain activity. They found that by using light stimulation in the way of flickering strobe lights combined with pulsating sound waves or even rhythmic physical movement, they could actually produce the same 'peak performance brain states' in ordinary people with no meditative experience at all. Over the last few years scientists and electronic engineers have used advanced technology to design a variety of mind machines that allow you to trigger these desired peak performance brain patterns at will!

Delta Waves – When you fall asleep delta waves become the dominant brain waves, ranging in frequency upto 4Hz.

With the possibilities of very advanced brain states and coherence, there exists evidence that individuals may be able to maintain consciousness while in a dominant delta state. This seems to be associated with certain deep trance-like states.

Within the delta state, your brain is triggered to release large quantities of human growth hormone (HGH). Professional body builders such as Frank Zane use mind machines immediately after a workout to promote the release of this powerful youth enhancing hormone.

UNLEASHING THE MAGIC OF THE ALPHA-STIM

Electrical stimulation of your brain at the proper frequency, waveform and current can quickly and sharply increase the levels of many neurotransmitters in your brain. The Alpha Stim is a small device that does just that. It has been used for many purposes from pain relief to peak performance in sports and business.

NATURAL STIMULATION FOR AN ENDORPHIN HIGH

The Alpha Stim is most widely used for pain relief. If you were to experience pain in your neck for example, when the area of the pain is electrically stimulated at appropriate frequencies and amplitudes, your body responds with a flood of endorphins, alleviating the pain and in some cases leading to complete recovery.

There is evidence that this kind of direct stimulation to the neurons of your brain (by the use of electrodes that clip to the ears) has a profound optimising and normalising effect on brain functioning. The use of the Alpha Stim and other forms of Cranial Electro-Stimulation (CES) facilitate a re-balancing of brain chemistry. CES seems to act directly on the neurons to stimulate the release of neuropeptides, such as the endorphins, and other neurotransmitters, such as norepinephrine and dopamine (associated with memory and learning), as well as serotonin, adrenocorticotropic (ACTH) and cholinesterase. Researchers have found CES effective in the treatment of depression, chronic pain, migraine headaches, treatment of learning disabilities and the treatment of children with cerebral palsy. It's now easy to…

BOOST BRAIN JUICES FOR LEARNING AND ECSTASY

When you stimulate the reward centres in your brain, you immediately experience more pleasure due to the increased flow of catecholamines (including norepinephrine and dopamine). These neurotransmitters have a very similar effect on your brain as cocaine. Norepinephrine is so pleasurable that if a drug could be created to stimulate it on its own, without dopamine, it would produce undiluted ecstasy. Now there's a thought!

Low frequency currents induced by external electrodes from machines such as the Alpha Stim can dramatically speed up the production of various neurotransmitters in your brain, with different brain juices being triggered by different frequencies and waveforms. For example, a 10-Hz signal boosts the production and turnover rate of serotonin.

Each brain centre generates impulses at a specific frequency based on the predominant neurotransmitters it secretes. In other words, your brain's internal communication system is based on frequency. When you send in waves of electrical energy at 10Hz for example, certain cells in the lower brain stem respond because they normally fire within that frequency range. As a result, particular mood-altering chemicals associated with that region will be released.

MEMORY'S MATE – GLUTAMATE

Glutamate isn't as well understood as most of the other neurotransmitters, but is definitely essential to the formation of memories and the retrieval of old ones.

When experiments were conducted on rabbits and rats, researchers discovered that the formation of memories was directly related to the number of glutamate receptors in the brain. By using electrical stimulation at specific rhythms and amplitudes, the levels of glutamate can be dramatically altered, playing an important role in the formation of memories. Low levels of glutamate in your brain generally indicate decreased cognitive function. Furthermore, glutamate can be especially helpful in brain longevity programs because it inhibits the chronic stress response and, consequently, the over production of cortisol.

BALANCING BRAIN BOOSTING JUICES
FOR PEAK PERFORMANCE

The very slow 0.5Hz waves of the Alpha Stim, can act as a toner resonating and stimulating every one of your brain cells, restoring harmony and balance. This is critical for the following reasons:

- Too much norepinephrine can lead to anxiety, tension, and hyperactivity. Too little can impair memory and cause depression.
- Too much acetylcholine leads to lethargy. Too little leads to weakness and hallucination.
- Too much serotonin causes hallucinations and sleep. Too little brings depression, aggression, and insomnia.

Your brain functions at its best when the various neurotransmitters are within their optimal range. You wouldn't want a stereo that blasts out base without any other frequency. You'd want balance. The same is true of your brain and your life.

By hooking yourself up to an Alpha Stim, you can activate your brain's learning pathways and enhance your ability to think, absorb new information, combine ideas in new and innovative ways, consolidate facts into memory, and recall information already stored in your brain. If you want to increase your ability to learn, think, create, imagine and explore, the only question is: How much and in what ways? Now, as you get excited at the infinite possibilities and potential, let me take you on another journey...

SENSORY PLEASURE WITH LIGHT-SOUND DEVICES

Modern scientific research into the effects of rhythmic light and sound began in the mid-1930s when scientists discovered that the electrical rhythms of the brain tended to assume the rhythm of a flashing light stimulus, a process called entrainment. For example, when they flashed a strobe light at a frequency of 10Hz into the eyes of a subject monitored by an electroencephalogram (EEG), the subject's brain waves tended to adopt a 10Hz frequency.

A flood of subsequent scientific research in the 1960s and 1970s revealed that such flicker effects at certain frequencies seemed to have amazing powers. Various scientists began discovering that photic-stimulation has a variety of beneficial effects, such as increasing IQ scores, enhancing intellectual functioning, and producing greater synchronisation between the two hemispheres of the brain. Other researchers found that the addition of rhythmic auditory signals dramatically increased the mind-enhancing effects. There is certainly more to these light-sound machines than meets the eye.

THE HEALING POWER OF 'FORGOTTEN BRAIN NUTRIENTS'

Light and sound are brain nutrients that stimulate the electrical energy in your brain. They energise and heal. Light, falling on the photoreceptors of your eye, is translated into electrical impulses, which then stimulates the entire brain, via the visual cortex and the hypothalamus. In addition, by stimulating the nerve endings in your ear (using pulses of sound), each pulse is translated into electrical impulses, which then stimulate the brain via the vestibular system, cerebellum, limbic system, and cortex. The most impressive way to send electrical impulses into your brain is by using the same rhythmic pulsation of electricity that naturally powers the brain cells. If light and sound are nutrients that enrich the brain with their electrical impulses, then the electrical impulses, if delivered in the correct form and at the correct intensity, are the purest nutrient. The Alpha Stim represents the best tool on the market to achieve this purity.

THE SOUND OF THE BINAURAL BEATS
HAS THE POWER TO ENTRAIN YOUR BRAIN

Robert Monroe, author of 'Journeys out of the Body', was the first person to really discover the power of stereo sound (played through stereo headphones) on the brain. For example, if you were to hear a signal of 200 cycles per second in your right ear, and a signal of 204 cycles per second in your left, the two hemispheres of your brain begin to function together and hear a phantom third signal. This signal, a binaural beat, is the difference in frequency between the two sound frequencies, in this case 4 cycles per second (4Hz). It isn't actually a beat, but an electrical signal created by both hemispheres of the brain when functioning harmoniously.

Monroe soon discovered that when precisely controlled tones are combined in the brain, the olivary nucleus begins to resonate sympathetically to this electrical signal/binaural beat. As this resonating/entrainment process begins to take place, signals are gradually sent into the cerebral cortex, mixing existing patterns of brain activity and causing profound state changes. By using certain frequencies, Monroe realised he could produce a unique and coherent brain state, known as hemispheric synchronisation.

ENDORPHINS, BINAURAL BEAT PATTERNS
AND BRAIN ENHANCEMENT

Scientists have also found that when the brain is exposed to alpha and theta binaural beat patterns, endorphins are released. Endorphins have a powerful strengthening effect on learning and memory, enhancing many mental functions, and have been known to reverse amnesia. Researcher David de Weid found that when rats were injected with endorphins their memory recall increased dramatically. 1977 Nobel Prize winner Andrew Schally found that when rats received injections of endorphins, their maze-running abilities immediately improved.

HOLOSYNC TECHNOLOGY – THE MOST REVOLUTIONARY
BINAURAL BEAT MIND/BODY DEVELOPMENT PROGRAM EVER!

Embedded on cassette/CD beneath soothing music and environmental sounds, the Holosync sound technology will lead you into the deeper alpha, theta and delta brain wave patterns. By providing more input to the brain than it can handle, the Holosync sound technology causes the brain to respond by reorganising itself at higher levels of function. By doing this the brain begins to handle the additional input, creating new neural pathways and establishing communication between parts of the brain that were not previously communicating. If you don't get your hands on The End® Personal Growth Through Technology program, developed by Bill Harris, you'll be missing out on one of the most powerful personal development tools in existence. To make it work, all you have to do is close your eyes and listen. It is an on-going personal development program utilising the Holosync® sound technology.

A recent study performed by Dr. Vincent Giampapa, M.D., of The Longevity Institute International and Vice President of The American Society of Anti-Ageing Medicine, revealed that the Holosync audio technology had dramatic effects on the production of cortisol, DHEA, and melatonin.

Although you know a lot about cortisol and DHEA, melatonin is an equally important hormone. It helps create a blissful night's sleep, and as you age, unless you take effective action, your body may make less of it. Sleep is critical because many important rejuvenating substances are created in the brain. Optimal sleep leads to a rich and fulfilling life. Poor sleeping habits can accelerate the ageing process.

In a before and after study of 19 people using Holosync audio technology, the following changes were noted in levels of melatonin, DHEA and cortisol:

- In just three days over 68% of the group had increases in DHEA levels, with an average increase of 43%! Several people had increases of 50%, 60%, and even 90%! A study published in the New England Journal of Medicine (12/11/86) found that a 100 microgram per decilitre increase in DHEA blood levels corresponded with a 48% drop in death from cardiovascular disease – and an overall 36 % reduction in death from all causes.
- Cortisol levels were down an average of 46.5%, with several people experiencing decreases of 70 or 80%!
- Melatonin levels increased by an average of 97.8%, with positive changes happening in over 73% of the people! Many had improvements of 100%, 200%, and even 300%!

♦ Contact Lifetools www.lifetools.com 01189 483444 for all your peak performance mind machines, including The End® Personal Growth Through Technology program.

ARE YOU READY FOR THE CHALLENGE?

The potential of the body and mind is limitless. Whether you find a brain gym in your local area or have to travel to find one, start investigating/investing in the following: PhotoReading by Paul Scheele, Light/Sound Machines, Cranial Electro-Stimulation (CES), EEG machines for biofeedback, binaural beat generator machines/CDs, motion machines, acoustic field generators, floatation tanks etc. I use an Alpha-Stim 100, a Mindlab Proteus and The End® Personal Growth Through Technology program. I get fantastic results in mood enhancement, whilst conditioning peak performance brain states. Let's recap on some important points:

♦ As you read let your awareness fall on your breathing...That's right...take a deep breath in...and when you are ready...Let it out fully...and evenly...relaxing as you do. Now, everyone knows that deep breathing has the potential to calm and relax you. But do you do this purposefully every day? Deep breathing will balance your chemistry as it alkalises your blood by removing carbon dioxide from your body. Remember carbon dioxide is acidic. As you breathe deeply, you take in more oxygen and exhale more carbon dioxide, whilst relieving stress.

♦ Shallow breathing results in poor oxygenation of the blood, increased stress levels, and decreased immunity. When you use mind machines, ensure you relax and breathe fully to get the most of your session.

♦ Studies have shown that with proper stimulation your brain can continue to grow, increasing your intelligence, even after 70, 80 or 90 years. Under the right conditions neurons can regenerate, suggesting that given the right type of stimulation your brain will continuously heal itself and replace lost cells, in much the same way as your skin can heal itself after it has been cut.

♦ One neuroscientist at the University of California at Los Angeles took specimens from over twenty human brains and analysed them under his microscope. He found a clear and definite relationship between the number of years of education and the length of the dendrites in the subjects brain. The more people had learned, the greater their dendritic length.

- Mind machines have been proven to improve both long-term and short-term memory. The Alpha Stim works by stimulating protein synthesis.

- For memories to become permanent in the brain, there has to be a process of nerve cell growth (protein synthesis) involving RNA (Ribonucleic acid), of which there is a greater concentration in your brain than anywhere else in your body. E3Live is an excellent source of RNA/DNA (nucleic acids).

- In several studies, subjects with learning disabilities have shown average increases in IQ over 20 or 30 points. Other research suggests that mind machines can dramatically boost the IQ of normal, healthy users.

- In a variety of settings, subjects using mind technology have learned more, learned faster, and proven more adept at learning difficult and complex material than ordinary subjects. Accelerated learning is encouraged since brain cells can forge new, richer interconnections.

- By actively reducing cortisol production with the use of mind machines you may be doing all that is necessary to enhance your immune system. This is because cortisol/stress inhibits delta 6 desaturase and eicosanoid production.

- Evidence shows that various mind machines can reduce levels of stress-related neuro-chemicals, dramatically reduce muscle tension, lower high blood pressure, slow heart rate, soothe jangled nerves, and quickly produce whole body levels of relaxation. All these benefits increase resistance to stress.

- The use of the Alpha Stim (Cranial Electro-Stimulation (CES)) restores homeostasis in the brain. CES seems to act directly on the neurons to stimulate the release of neuropeptides, including endorphins, norepinephrine, dopamine, serotonin, adrenocorticotropic (ACTH) and cholinesterase.

- A 10Hz signal boosts the production and turnover rate of serotonin. Each brain centre generates impulses at a specific frequency based on the predominant neurotransmitters it secretes. In other words, the brain's internal communication system is based on frequency.

- By using electrical stimulation at specific rhythms and amplitudes to stimulate the brain, levels of glutamate can be dramatically altered, playing an important role in the formation of memory. A low level of glutamate in your brain indicates a decrease in cognitive function.

- By hooking yourself up to an Alpha Stim, you can activate your brain's learning pathways and enhance your ability to think, absorb new information, combine ideas in new innovative ways, consolidate facts into memory, and recall information in your brain.

♦ A flood of scientific research in the 1960s and 1970s revealed that flicker effects at certain frequencies seemed to have amazing powers on the brain. Subjects experienced increased IQ scores, enhanced intellectual functioning, and greater synchronisation between the two hemispheres of the brain. Other researchers found that the addition of rhythmic auditory signals dramatically increased the mind-enhancing effects. There is more to light/sound machines than meets the eye.

It's up to you to take this technology as far as you can. Combine it with a nutritional plan that supplies your brain and body with vibrancy and you'll have an awesome future in front of you. Whether you're in sports, business or simply want to learn something new – Mind machines must play a part in your daily routine!

THE RAW PERFECTION EVALUATION
Have you experimented with mind machines yet?
Have you purchased a mind machine yet?
Do you use your mind machine daily for peak
performance/relaxation?

CHAPTER 13

DEVELOPING A BRAIN LIKE EINSTEIN: THE POWER OF ENRICHMENT

Although I'm sure you are excited about getting your hands on a mind machine, let me take you back in time – back in time when neuroscience was in its infancy. Back in time when brain science involved a laboratory and a group of rats! I'm not a great advocate of animal experimentation, but the results from these studies will certainly open your mind and expand your awareness to the unlimited power that resides within all of us.

A BRIEF HISTORY OF FINDINGS: THE SECRETS EINSTEIN LEFT BEHIND

In the 1980s, Dr Marion Diamond, Neuroanatomist and leading expert in the area of brain research, was given the honour of dissecting and studying the brain of Albert Einstein. At the time, many of the members of the neurological sciences were eager to find out if the brains of geniuses had any distinguishing characteristics that separated them from so-called 'average' people.

When Einstein was alive, he used to explain that when he was in deep thought or day dreaming, his thoughts were simply a combination of 'certain signs and more or less clear images.' He used to think visually primarily, and said that words played no part in the process. Using this to her advantage, Dr Diamond chose to carefully examine the sections of Einstein's brain that were responsible for vivid imagery and abstract reasoning. These areas are known as the superior prefrontal and inferior parietal lobes.

To ensure her findings were as credible as possible, Diamond compared the results against a control group of brains, all of which were taken from intellectually average men, who had also died at age 76, like Einstein. What Dr Diamond discovered was that each of the brains, including Einstein's was almost physically identical, except for one distinguishing feature – The appearance of Area 39.

EXERCISE LIKE EINSTEIN – STIMULATE GLIAL CELLS AND IMPROVE THE FUNCTION OF AREA 39

The one distinguishing feature that made Einstein's brain stand out from the rest was the abundance of a particular type of cell in an area of his brain known as Area 39. If a person has lesions in Area 39, they have great difficulties with abstract imagery, memory, attention, and self-awareness, whilst showing a difficulty in integrating visual, auditory and kinaesthetic input. With problems in Area 39, a person can lose most of their higher intellect and display an inability to read, recognise letters, spell or do calculations.

The name of the cell that was in great abundance in Area 39 was the glial cell. Many people thought that glial cells were thinking cells, but it was discovered that they are actually 'house keeping' cells. Due to the intensity of Einstein's thinking, Area 39 needed a great deal of metabolic support, resulting in the accumulation of these cells, enlarging Einstein's Area 39.

Many people used to think Einstein was a 'born genius', with an efficient brain, but research is now proving that anyone can enlarge areas of their brain if they are willing to mentally exercise it. Einstein created his own genius, and you can do the same! The research continued, leading to...

MORE FINDINGS, MORE POTENTIAL, MORE EXCITEMENT

Biological Psychologists Mark Rosenzweig and colleagues at the University of California performed various experiments on rats in order to explore brain function. They had already discovered that the reason rats conquer mazes at different speeds is due to their learning ability. This ability to learn is primarily affected by a brain enzyme known as acetylcholinesterase (AChE). After various maze tests they found that the higher the level of AChE in the brain, the faster the rat learned. What they didn't know was whether this enzyme could be manipulated through stimulation, or whether its production was simply down to genetics. They decided to conduct a series of experiments. They took a group of genetically equal rats and divided them into three groups.

1. Group one was put in a standard environment – a mesh cage.
2. Group two was put in isolation. Each rat was subjected to a cage with three opaque walls, dim lights, little noise, minimal stimulation, and no chance to interact with other rats. This was the impoverished environment.
3. Group three was raised in play groups of ten to twelve rats, in large, well-lit, multi-levelled cages filled with swings, slides, ladders, bridges, an assortment of toys, frequently changing stimuli, and a variety of challengers. This was called the enriched environment, suggesting you can...

STIMULATE AChE BY ENRICHING YOUR LIFE

After certain periods of time ranging from days to a number of months, the brains of the rats were removed and analysed. To their astonishment, researchers discovered that the rats raised in the enriched environment showed higher levels of AChE activity in their brain cortex than the rats raised in the standard and impoverished environments. (The cerebral cortex is a layer of nerve cells, where much of the thinking and higher intellectual activity of the brain takes place.) They found that cortical AChE activity isn't a fixed individual characteristic, but could be altered by experience!

Since AChE activity was directly linked to their ability to learn and process information, the rats in the enriched environment had developed a greater ability to learn and had become smarter than the other rats. Experience had altered intelligence. Now is the time to...

STIMULATE YOUR SENSES
AND PUT WEIGHT ON WHERE IT COUNTS!

As you might imagine, the researchers were more than just a little startled. What they accidentally stumbled across next was more than just remarkable, it challenged everything they believed about the brain up until that point. The way they measured AChE was by 'enzymatic activity per unit of tissue weight'. To do this they weighed brain samples, so they could measure chemical activity per unit of tissue weight. After two years of doing this they noticed that the actual weight of the brain samples also changed, the cortex of the rats in the enriched-environment had actually become heavier than the cortex of the other rats! Stimulating experiences had caused the rats' brains to grow. This finding sparked off a frenzy of studies and research that resulted in some groundbreaking findings in the field of neuroscience. In all cases, the rats raised in the enriched environment showed:

♦ An increase in the thickness and size of individual neurons in the cortex.
♦ An increase in protein levels, in alignment with increases in cortical weight. This proved that it was tissue growth and not an increased fluid level that was causing the weight gain.
♦ An increase in the amount of dendritic branching. Imagine your hand is the cell body of the neuron and your fingers are the dendrites. With use and enriched environments your brain develops more branching. The nerve cells are designed to receive stimulation, so an increase in dendritic branching means an increase in possible connections.
♦ An increased number of dendritic spines per unit length of dendrite. The spines are the thousands of small projections that cover the surface of dendrites. Each one marking the site of a synapse, the point where another neuron makes a junction with this neuron. With an increase in the number of spines there exists a greater potential for interconnection between neurons.
♦ Increases in the number of synapses and in the size of synaptic contact areas. Synapses are the spots where different neurons are connected and by means of which communication amongst neurons takes place. By increasing their number and size, you increase the richness of communication in the cortex.

- An increase in the ratio between the weight of the cortex and the weight of the rest of the brain. The enriched environment is beneficial to the area that primarily controls thinking, learning and memory.
- A 15% increase in the number of glial cells. Out of all the cells in the brain these are the most numerous. They act like glue and hold together, support and nourish the brain neurons. They also act as guides for neural growth, assist in learning and also have a communicating network of their own. The message is clear...

ENRICH YOUR LIFE WITH AN ENRICHED ENVIRONMENT

Brain experiments were becoming increasingly fascinating and the potential of the brain – limitless. Dr Diamond continued her studies of Area 39. She was curious to find out whether it was the simple act of thinking that caused the unusual growth and she designed an experiment to test her theory. To begin with she built two totally different environments. The first one was a small box with nothing in it. The second one was filled with a variety of toys and games. Into the bare box Dr Diamond placed one rat and her three offspring. Into the second box she placed three female rats, with three offspring each.

Dr Diamond wasn't surprised to find that when the rats died, those that had spent their lives in the enriched environment had a 16% larger Area 39 than in the other rats. What she didn't expect to find was that other areas of their brains had also increased in size, by about 10%. She went on to find that this worked just as successfully with elderly rats, proving it's never to late to challenge and stimulate yourself. Now is the time for the critical question:

ARE YOU LIVING IN AN IMPOVERISHED ENVIRONMENT?

If you are still not sold on the idea of mentally stimulating yourself, think about this: Dr Diamond discovered that without enough thought provoking toys and an environment to match, the brains of rats could actually shrink. Could this be the reason for age-associated memory decline and cognitive impairment? Having been raised in a mentally impoverished environment, the dorsal cortex of the rats' brain shrunk by 9% and the entohorinal cortex, which is associated to memory, shrunk by 25%. It's up to you to stimulate yourself and...

DEVELOP WISDOM BY CREATING MORE
SIX SIDED DENDRITES

To delve even deeper into the intricacies of neuron development, Dr Diamond found that highly developed neurons responded better to enriched environments than less developed ones. During the developmental process, neurons reach out to other neurons with branch-like dendrites. As new information is assimilated, dendrites keep sending out new branches, and those branches send out more branches again. Dr Diamond discovered that the first, second, third, forth and fifth dendrite didn't grow any longer even though exposed to an enriched environment, but the sixth branch did.

She explains that, "Whether we are young or old, we can continue to learn. The brain can change at any age. We began with a nerve cell, which starts in the embryo as just a sort of sphere. It sends its first branch out just to overcome ignorance. As it reaches out, it is gathering knowledge and it is becoming creative. Then we become a little more idealistic, generous, and altruistic; but it is our six-sided dendrites which give us wisdom."

CREATE SUPER ENRICHMENT – TODAY!

To follow these amazing findings, Argentinean researchers created a super-enriched environment and to their surprise found that it caused as much brain growth in four days as took place in thirty days in the ordinary enriched environments.

A short while later they found that four daily one-hour periods of enriched exposure significantly increased cortical growth. Then they went on to find that four daily exposures to an enriched environment, of only ten minutes, brought about significant increases in cortical weight! Other investigators found that a single forty-five minute session (where rats had to learn to choose various lighted alleys to avoid a nasty shock) resulted in significant brain changes, such as increases in the number and shape of some synapses. It got to the point where even short exposures to an enriched environment produced significant and long lasting effects on the cortex, sometimes within seconds of sensory stimulation! That's right – seconds!

HELPING THE AGED THROUGH STIMULATION

How would you describe nursing homes, hospitals and retirement homes? Would you call them enriched environments or impoverished environments? Obviously they have their uses, and in some cases are certainly the best option. Is it also possible to see them as the equivalent to 'impoverished environments'? Would it be fair to compare the lives of the elderly in retirement homes to the lives of rats who were placed in an impoverished environment, alone, cut off from challenges, change, companionship, and other sensory/intellectual stimulation. The rats experienced stunted brain growth and accompanying mental dullness/retardation. Could this also be one of the main reasons why humans placed in similarly impoverished environments lose their ability to think?

STIMULATE THE AGED AND REVERSE THE EFFECTS OF IMPOVERISHED ENVIRONMENTS

What is promising is that if the rats were taken out of their impoverished environments and placed in an enriched environment, the conditions of mental deterioration reverse almost immediately. For example, in one study, rats were isolated for 535 days until they reached middle age. Then they were presented with an enriched environment and quickly responded with rapid brain growth. This demonstrates one thing: It is never too late to make changes, and allow sharp and rapid development to be your birthright, no matter how dull the stimulation has been in the past.

BEGIN TO VALUE THE UNKNOWN AND WRESTLE WITH ENRICHMENT

The point is simple. If you continue to assimilate new information, if you continue to tackle challenges, if you continue to welcome change and new unpredictable experiences, you are assuring mental enhancement and complete mental health. To provide yourself with an enriched environment, your brain will continue to weave an ever richer, subtler and a more complex tapestry of neural connections, leading to increasing numbers of possible brain states. It is easy to see why communities such as the Hunzas who not only eat very healthfully but also challenge themselves physically and mentally, live incredibly long lives compared to most people in Western civilisation. The evidence indicates that it is not age that brings wisdom, but enriched environments.

Like the rats placed in the super-enriched environment (that showed as much brain growth in four hours, as the rats in the 'enriched environment' showed in a month), there exists a human equivalent. Mind machines – They subject the brain to intense amounts of stimulation and thus force-feed enrichment to your neurons, alter brain-wave activity, and trigger rapid brain growth.

HIGH PERFORMANCE, OPTIMAL PERFORMANCE, EXTRA-ORDINARY PERFORMANCE

The implications of these recent discoveries are quite clear: the brain is much more powerful, capable, and complex than had previously been imagined. What you think of as 'normal intelligence' is probably just a pale shadow of the brain's actual powers and faculties. Brain function can be substantially improved, provided the brain receives the right type of stimulation. Many mind machines are designed for exactly that, to increase mental power and stimulate actual growth of the physical brain. You now stand at a crossroads where you can make one of the most important decisions of your life...

GAZE INTO THE FUTURE AND DREAM OF THE INFINITE POSSIBILITIES

Energy and matter are constantly flowing into your brain in the form of light, sound, sensations, information, oxygen and nutrients from your bloodstream. Whilst your brain is only about 2% of total body weight, it uses more than 20% of all oxygen taken into your body, making it the most prodigious energy consumer.

RAW PERFECTION begins with the premise that in order to achieve greater than normal potential, and develop higher than ordinary capabilities, you must have energy. By operating your physiology optimally you set the foundation for a life of pleasure and discovery. Even though the mind machines I talk about have been used to stimulate the brains of people with a variety of neurological problems, including Down's Syndrome, mental retardation, and learning disabilities, think of them as your key to the doorway of peak performance. Extraordinary performance awaits you, giving you the chance to evolve as much as you choose through learning, growth and enriched experience. Remember the ultimate creative capacity of the brain may be, for all practical purposes, infinite.

ARE YOU READY FOR THE CHALLENGE?

When you've built incredible health and energy levels, your body wil require less sleep, leaving you with more time on your hands. You'll begir to avoid countless hours of mind numbing television as you search fo ways to exercise your mind and body. Whatever you choose to stimulat your higher thought processes, expect the kind of mental development tha will serve your mind and emotions for the rest of your life. Let's recap:

♦ Einstein had a far greater abundance of a particular type of cell in ar area of his brain known as Area 39. People with lesions in Area 39 have great difficulties with abstract imagery, memory, attention, and self-awareness, whilst showing a difficulty in integrating visual, auditory and kinaesthetic input. It's a very highly evolved area of the brain.

♦ Einstein spent many hours in deep thought, which is why Area 39 needed a great deal of metabolic support. Glial cells (house keeping cells) were abundant in this area of his brain, which accounted for its above average size.

♦ Create your own enriched environment with challenges and puzzles that stimulate you to think. Set yourself goals. Physical, mental, emotional, and even spiritual. When rats are raised in large, well-lit, multileveled cages, filled with swings, slides, ladders, bridges, an assortment of toys, they benefit from enrichment. Their brains mirror this.

♦ The ability to learn is primarily affected by a brain enzyme known as acetylcholinesterase (AChE). After various maze tests researchers found that rats with higher levels of AChE learned better than those with low levels. Cortical AChE activity isn't a fixed individual characteristic. You can alter it by stimulation!

♦ Stimulate your senses and put weight on where it counts. You can increase the thickness and size of individual neurons in the cortex of your brain, increase the amount of dendritic branching, increase the number of dendritic spines per unit length of a dendrite, increase the number of synapses and the size of synaptic contact areas and increase the ratio between the weight of the cortex and the weight of the rest of the brain. An enriched environment is beneficial to the area that primarily controls thinking, learning and memory.

♦ Dr Diamond discovered that the first, second, third, forth and fifth dendrites didn't grow any longer even though exposed to an enriched environment, but the sixth branch did.

♦ Stimulate the aged and reverse the effects of impoverished environments. Enriched environments have been used to reverse mental deterioration in elderly rats, whilst simultaneously causing brain growth. Everyone has the potential to make changes, no matter how dull the stimulation has been in the past.

♦ Mind machines subject the brain to intense amounts of stimulation and thus force-feed enrichment to your neurons and trigger rapid brain growth.

♦ One hour of reading in your chosen field each day will make you an authority in that field in 3 years, a national authority in that field in 5 years, and an international authority in that field in 7 years. Invest in Paul Scheele's PhotoReading Personal Learning Course from www.lifetools.com. When you read about it you'll know why!

Many people stop learning when they leave school. They develop a phobia of books and of the unfamiliar. Let this be someone else, not you! Embrace the unknown and expand your mind. What have you always wanted to learn or master? Maybe you've always wanted to learn to play a musical instrument? Maybe you've always wanted to learn how to play golf, tennis, squash or snooker? Maybe you've always wanted to increase your memory and IQ? Whatever ignites the flame of desire within you, begin today. Forget about results and enjoy getting lose within the activity. The joy and development comes in the doing, not the outcome! If you find yourself struggling, it's because your brain is figuring out a way for you to succeed. Be patient, persist, and you will.

The choice is yours: A dull brain and a lifeless body, or a brain that is charged with electricity, searching for challenge, enrichment and novelty.

THE RAW PERFECTION EVALUATION:
Do you challenge yourself and stimulate your brain frequently?
Do you have a ferocious desire to learn?

Every day, millions of people rely on chocolate, coffee, cakes and biscuits to increase the stimulation in their lives, compromising the performance of their body and brain. They wonder why they can't get motivated, become inspired or reach any level of creativity. Many people live lives of quiet desperation, whilst their mind and emotions remain out of control.

CHAPTER 14

FOOD FOR THOUGHT:
FEEDING YOUR NEUROTRANSMITTERS

Just stop for a moment and flick through this chapter. At first glance what you are about to discover may seem quite complex, but the distinctions that await you are critical in completing your understanding of RAW PERFECTION.

Neurotransmitters are communicators of information. Each and every one of them has a profound and important impact upon your life. Without them you'd lose the ability to think, experience emotions, process information, and basically stay alive. They are critical to memory, focus, learning, energy, happiness etc. and controlling them is ultimately down to what you eat and when. It's up to you to take control and learn how to balance them. Food is the raw material, you are the scientist and your brain is the laboratory.

BALANCING THE NEUROTRANSMITTERS
AND FEELING GREAT

As you cruise through the rest of this chapter, take a brief look at what you're about to learn:

1. Endorphins: The Keys To Paradise
2. Acetylcholine: The Essential Memory Nutrient
3. Norepinephrine: The Key To Staying Sharp And Alert
4. Dopamine/Serotonin: The Critical Neurotransmitter Axis
5. Nitric Oxide: Memory Formation And Erections

CONTROL YOUR BRAIN CHEMISTRY
AND CONTROL YOUR LIFE

The message of this chapter is simple: Food affects your brain chemistry, and your brain chemistry affects your mood. When your brain is balanced chemically, you will feel a sense of peace and calmness, whilst awakening your higher mind.

Sarah Leibowitz, Ph.D., one of the world's leading experts on the neurobiology of obesity, has demonstrated that various diets and various foods create very powerful changes in the brain.

The high fat/high carbohydrate 'junk food' diet alters the composition of the brain, stripping it of the neurotransmitters that foster a positive mood. This diet also dramatically increases the production of the hormones that cause overeating and bingeing. The brain of an obese person is chemically different from that of a thin person, and the habits that lead to obesity create a devastating downward spiral causing a biologically altered, inferior brain structure! The chain of events that lead to the downward spiral begins when the abuser creates a pleasurable association towards recreational/junk foods. Unfortunately, after the abuser has experienced the brief euphoric feeling that 'recreational food' supplies, they experience a debilitating 'physical low', caused by low blood sugar levels, unconsciously encouraging another fix.

Did you know that there are 40 million people in the U.S. reported as clinically depressed? The above conditions are all a result of a biologically altered brain, resulting from poor nutrition.

THE WORST CASE SCENARIO:
REFINED CARBOHYDRATES AND CRIME

Many of the foods served in jails include the following: sugar, coffee, white flour, margarine, mashed potatoes, quartered tomatoes, white bread, iceberg lettuce, pork chops, beef, and chicken. How is a brain supposed to operate well if it isn't fed right? Your brain is created daily from the food you eat, and your brain effects your behaviour. It's a basic law of behavioural biology!

To illustrate the power of food to control behaviour, a small study was carried out with inmates of a particular jail. It concluded that if you teach them to eat foods that help maintain stable blood sugar levels, only 20% return to crime, instead of the usual 80%. Researchers suggested that 90% of violent crimes are committed when the individual is suffering from low blood glucose (hypoglycaemia).

A brain deprived of its required fuel, shifts from higher cortical functions (conceptual, socially acceptable, knowing right from wrong) to lizard brain (fight or flight) functions. When the brain is in this state, even a minor stimulus can trigger off 'fight or flight' behaviour. Good nutrition protects the brain from entering 'fight or flight' mode, allowing it to function at a higher cortical level.

1 - ENDORPHINS: THE KEYS TO PARADISE

Although endorphins are not technically neurotransmitters, their effects are similar. They were discovered in the 1970s and are your body's own opiates. When you think of opiates you probably think of drugs such as heroin, morphine and opium don't you? But did you realise that the act of eating 'junk food' also supplies a hit of opiates to your brain?

People love to eat burgers and chips because they stimulate a short-lived endorphin 'high'. They are stimulating their brain with a shot of opiates. When someone injects heroin, they also stimulate their brain with a shot of opiates. So what's the difference? Dosage!

Think about it. Why is chocolate cake is a billion-pound industry? There's no logical reason to buy it. It's not nutritious. It makes you fat. It screws up your metabolism. And it's expensive. The only reason to buy it is because it feels so good to eat it!

In fact, the easiest way to make more endorphins in the short-term is by eating refined sugars and starches such as white flour breads, cereals, and pastas. But as you know these foods cause hormonal chaos on many levels.

WHY IS THERE SUCH A CURIOUS ATTRACTION BETWEEN HUMANS AND OPIATES?

Answer: Because opiates have a molecular structure similar to endorphin molecules, and the glucose receptor is closely associated with the endorphin system.

Although highly sophisticated, your brain was never designed to deal with sugar overload, but due to mass production of recreational convenience foods, sugar/carbohydrate addiction is now one of the most deadly addictions of all, along with smoking, alcoholism and drug abuse. Just as recreational drugs cause depression, low self-esteem, anxiety, and a myriad of other less than empowering states, the chronic use of food as a recreational drug also has this effect.

RECREATIONAL FOOD ABUSE CAUSES MORE DEATHS THAN RECREATIONAL DRUG ABUSE

In America 'junk food' is consumed at a frightening rate and 70% of all deaths in the U.S. can be linked to 'junk food' abuse. It is an addiction that is taking over the world. The addictive components of tea, coffee, chocolate and cocoa are all chemically related to 'speed' (amphetamine).

Even though cocaine and heroin (two of the most deadly drugs) are responsible for causing misery amongst many of their abusers, they don't account for anywhere near the same number of deaths associated with poor nutritional habits. Cocaine and heroin kill approximately 3000 people per year, 1500 each.

The problem with recreational convenience food is that it is often loaded with sugar, toxins and cooked fats. It causes massive increases in insulin, and simultaneous increases in body fat and toxicity. The endorphins that are released whilst eating these 'junk foods', immediately diminish and create more cravings, until another shot of opiates hits the brain, encouraging the binge cycle. There aren't a lot of fat heroin addicts, but there are plenty of fat endorphin addicts. Food is the key to controlling your overall mood and emotions.

ACCESSING A FLOOD OF MOOD ENHANCING NEUROCHEMICALS WITH MIND MACHINES

Another function of endorphins is to shield you from the psychological and physical effects of extreme stress. As stress mounts, your endorphins counteract some of the effects of the stress response, and sometimes in an effort to alleviate stress and stimulate a quick endorphin 'boost', many people reach for recreational/junk food.

Do you want a better way to produce states of euphoria, energy, comfort, relaxation and joy, rather than turning to food? Mind machines may be the answer for you. I've used them to maintain balance when a hectic work schedule presents itself. If you are reading this book with the intention of losing unwanted fat, you need to break the habit of using recreational foods to activate your natural reward system. I recommend mind machines as a powerful alternative.

The habit of choosing food to alter your state is nothing but a calculated act of neurochemical self-adjustment. Just as a heroin addict is adjusting his or her neurochemical balance by consuming an endorphin substitute, many people use food to trigger the release of endorphins. These unconscious acts cause our brains to release the same neurochemicals associated with motherly love, happiness, comfort, and fulfilment, but there are many downsides.

When you use mind technology, you immediately produce rapid alterations in brain chemistry, restoring the natural balance of pleasure neurochemicals depleted by food or substance abuse. Simultaneously you strengthen and exercise the pleasure pathways within your brain. What a deal!

EUPHORIA IN THE WOMB

Your first experience of 'endorphin euphoria' was in your mother's womb. When she was pregnant she would have been producing levels of endorphins at least eight times higher than normal! If you were breastfed you would have benefited from the blissful effects of endorphins present in your mother's milk. Studies have shown that when babies are separated from their mothers, they display high levels of anxiety. If, however, the synthetic equivalent of endorphins is fed to them their anxiety disappears and they return to their blissful state. Endorphins alleviate anxiety and act as a substitute for motherly love and nourishment. Make sure you choose wisely where you get your next fix!

HOW TO BOOST ENDORPHINS NATURALLY

So, you've had enough of using artificial means to stimulate your brain. You want to produce more endorphins on a consistent basis using natural measures. The answer: Exercise. A mere thirty minutes or more of exercise will give you the same endorphin boost as a chocolate bar, but it will last all day, not just a few seconds. The best time to workout is in the morning, especially if you want to start your day on an endorphin high.

Endorphins have numerous roles within the body but essentially exist to bring you pleasure. Pleasure in the presence of pain, pleasure to alleviate stress, pleasure to reward you, pleasure to enhance or suppress memories and pleasure to determine what information you filter into your brain. If you want to learn massive amounts of information, then ensure you are in an environment that is incredibly pleasurable. It is a scientific fact that when your endorphins are flowing, information is more easily assimilated. Mind machines can cause endorphin levels to rise, which is why learning can be easier when you use the power of these machines. Endorphins encourage you to continue what you're doing; they stimulate interest, increase your focus, and help you develop laser-like concentration. Use raw plant food, exercise and mind machines to get the most out of your body, mind and life. Let's re-cap:

- The natural euphoric high that is associated with running is caused by an increase flow of endorphins in the brain.
- Endorphins are critical in pain reduction, and are released in response to virtually any kind of significant physical or emotional stress.
- Endorphins encourage you to continue what you're doing. They stimulate interest, focus, and concentration. Mind machines can cause endorphin levels to rise, which is why learning can be easier when you use the power of these machines.
- People love to eat chocolate because it stimulates a short-lived endorphin 'high'. However, a mere thirty minutes or more of exercise will give you the same boost that will last all day, not just a matter of seconds. Workout in the morning and you'll feel great all day.
- Endorphins exist to bring you pleasure. Pleasure in the presence of pain,

pleasure to alleviate stress, pleasure to reward you, pleasure to enhance/suppress memories and pleasure to determine what information you filter into your brain.

♦ By using mind machines, you'll immediately begin to produce rapid alterations in brain chemistry, restoring the natural balance of pleasure neurochemicals depleted by food or substance abuse, whilst simultaneously strengthening and exercising the pleasure pathway within your brain. What a deal!

♦ If you want to learn massive amounts of information, ensure you are in an environment that is incredibly pleasurable. Use mind machines to get your endorphin juices flowing and information will become more easily assimilated. And to enhance the process of information assimilation even more, embrace...

2 - THE ESSENTIAL MEMORY NUTRIENT –
ACETYLCHOLINE

In the middle of the 20th Century, scientists discovered that acetylcholine is the most abundant neurotransmitter in the brain. Essential to higher mental processes such as learning and memory, acetylcholine has adopted the reputation of 'superstar neurotransmitter of memory and thought.' It is particularly concentrated in the hippocampus, the structure essential to the formation and recall of long-term memories. The power of this neurotransmitter is such that if you have a poor memory, but are too young to be suffering from memory impairment associated with old age, you've probably just a simple acetylcholine deficit. Acetylcholine helps neurons in the cortex retain the imprint of incoming information.

Even the confusion and loss of memory associated with Alzheimer's disease has now been linked in part to a lack of acetylcholine in certain areas of the brain. If however, acetylcholine is injected into those areas, or the subjects are given acetylcholine-boosting drugs, sufferers of the disease respond with dramatic gains in memory and other mental abilities. It's up to you to...

INCREASE ACETYLCHOLINE
AND INCREASE YOUR BRAIN POWER

If you want to improve your memory, learning ability and intelligence, and develop a mind that can focus like a laser, ensure you maintain optimal brain levels of acetylcholine. Studies of normal subjects show significant increases in scores on memory tests when given substances that increase the amount of acetylcholine in their brain. The important question:

WHAT ARE THESE SUBSTANCES THAT INCREASE THE MEMORY MOLECULE?

Acetylcholine is produced within neurons by a complicated chemical process that requires oxygen, glucose, and the action of an enzyme, dependent on vitamin B5 and choline. The combination of B5 and choline is incredibly effective in enhancing memory and mental performance.

The Central American University Report (1994) on malnourished grammar school children stated that academic results and exam scores improved tremendously after trials of wild blue-green algae were administered. E3Live has a unique energy that has an affinity to improving brain function. Clinical research shows that AFA algae balances EEG readings and improves central nervous functioning. In addition to consuming E3Live, eat more sprouted nuts and seeds, green leafy vegetables and include sprouted Soybeans in your daily nutritional routine. In the process of germination, the desirable phosphorus compounds such as lecithin increase dramatically.

WHETHER IT'S AN INCREASE IN MEMORY OR A CLEARER STATE OF MIND, CHOLINE IS THE KEY

Fortunately the brain has the ability to absorb choline very rapidly and in times of stress, it has been proven that choline can provide an immediate boost to brain power. If you are studying or have a test or exam, a dose of choline is vital and will allow your brain to operate at its very best. Studies have shown that choline can also improve overall mental functioning and thought transmission, strengthening neurons in the memory centre of your brain. To illustrate this point, students at the Massachusetts Institute of Technology who took choline found they could learn longer lists of words and could remember better. Many people who take choline state that they have a clearer perception and feel that their overall mental functioning is enhanced. UC Berkeley researcher Mark Rosenzweig has shown a direct connection between acetylcholine and intelligence.

Acetylcholine also helps perform many functions outside the brain. For example if you read the Arnold Schwarzenegger Encyclopaedia of Body Building, you'll find that Arnold himself used lecithin (also rich in choline), in his early days of training, helping to build high levels of acetylcholine in his body and thus enhance the action of the nerve cells in his muscles to trigger muscle action. If it's good enough for Arnie then it's good enough for you! If you are an athlete...

USE SOY AND E3LIVE TO PREVENT THE POTENTIAL HAZARDS OF ENDURANCE EVENTS

When the blood profiles of marathon runners were studied, choline levels fluctuated dramatically. Researcher Richard Wurtman discovered that after 26 miles of running, choline levels drop by a staggering 40%. Studies also show that swimmers are able to swim for longer (without the perils of muscle fatigue) when choline is introduced into their diet. By consuming E3Live on a daily basis and eating sprouted Soybeans, you'll increase your choline levels dramatically.

MANIPULATE THE CHEMISTRY OF YOUR BRAIN AND UNLEASH SUPER-INTELLIGENCE

As your diet changes, so does the chemistry of your brain, leaving it up to you to make the right choices. Treat acetylcholine as the foundation of your memory and brainpower and do all you can to eat foods that stimulate its production. Let's re-cap:

- Acetylcholine has adopted the reputation of 'superstar neurotransmitter of memory and thought'.
- Acetylcholine helps neurons in the cortex retain the imprint of incoming information.
- A simple acetylcholine deficit is often the answer if you have a poor memory, but too young to be suffering from memory impairment associated with old age.
- Even the confusion and loss of memory associated with Alzheimer's disease has now been linked to a lack of acetylcholine in certain areas of the brain. If however, acetylcholine is injected into those areas, or the

subjects are given acetylcholine-boosting drugs, sufferers of the disease respond with dramatic gains in memory and other mental abilities.

♦ Keep brain levels of acetylcholine optimal and you'll help prevent memory loss and cognitive dysfunction.

♦ Studies of normal subjects show significant increases in scores on memory tests when given substances that increase the amount of acetylcholine in their brain.

♦ Acetylcholine is produced within neurons by a complicated chemical process that requires oxygen, glucose, and choline (the primary ingredient of lecithin).

♦ The combination of B5 and choline has proved effective in enhancing memory and mental performance.

♦ There is nothing difficult about restoring acetylcholine to normal levels, simply eat more greens. A chlorophyll-based 'green drink' will supply about 2g of lecithin per serving. A recommended dose would be approximately 2-3g four times daily, for a total daily dosage of approximately 8-12g. Eat, juice and blend your greens and consume E3Live/wheatgrass juice daily.

♦ Fortunately the brain has the ability to absorb choline very rapidly and in times of stress, it has been proven that choline can provide an immediate boost to brain power. When studying or taking exams ensure you increase your intake of greens. A simple dose will allow your brain to operate at peak levels of functioning, but what good is laser like memory if your mind is dull and listless? Welcome...

3 – NOREPINEPHRINE:
THE KEY TO STAYING SHARP AND ALERT

Norepinephrine (NE) is a hormone that also functions as a neurotransmitter. It has an arousing, sharpening effect on the brain causing incredible alertness. NE is also vital in helping carry memories from short-term storage in the hippocampus to long-term storage in the neocortex.

Did you ever wonder why certain memories (especially ones that you experienced at moments of heightened arousal), remain vivid in your mind? That's NE in action. Whether it's great joy, intense fear, crisis, or love, when you're riding the wave of an adrenaline rush the memories are 'indelibly burned' into your memory. As mentioned earlier, however, too much norepinephrine can prevent the formation of new memories, and can interfere with rational thought and decision making, highlighting…

THE DANGERS AND EFFECTS OF THE DRUG 'SPEED'

NE plays a key role in memory and learning. The drug amphetamine (also known as speed) has a structure similar to NE, and when consumed increases the effects of NE in the brain. Although the drug is very dangerous with many side effects, students have often favoured it when cramming for exams. By eliminating the action of the adrenal glands and preventing the arousing effects, amphetamine stimulates a rapid increase in NE, enhancing the learning and memory processes. This unnatural state of intense mental alertness, allows large amounts of information to be absorbed and remembered (although many students use it to dance until dawn rather than cram for exams). But be warned, 'speed' can cause permanent brain damage and is often purchased illegally, having been mixed/cut with other toxic substances.

NE also governs your sleep patterns. Too much NE makes it almost impossible to fall asleep, which is why those who take 'speed' can often be found burning the midnight oil.

THE DANGERS OF THE DIET PILL ILLUSION

Did you know that many diet pills have been taken off the market because they contained amphetamine? The pills appeared to be useful to begin with because they stimulate NE which kills the appetite, causes insulin levels to drop, and fat to be burned as fuel. The only problem is that the body responds as if there is a famine and enters a survival/storage mode. The pills work well to cause an increase in metabolism, but at the expense of upsetting the body's natural rhythm. Drugs for weight loss are dangerous and unnecessary! If you are tempted to buy slimming pills, imagine yourself a year from now even fatter and more tired than you've ever been as you try to hold onto a life that is slipping away. I hope my point is clear, use food as your drug and…

ACCESS YOUR OWN PURE NOREPINEPHRINE

Even though pure amphetamine is powerful, pure NE is superior in every way. Studies have concluded that when NE levels in the brain are reduced, memory and learning abilities drop dramatically. Cornell researchers found that by inhibiting the synthesis of NE in rats' brains, they interrupted their overall ability to remember for more than twenty-four hours.

Studies now show that if you increase NE levels in your brain, memory and learning ability increase dramatically. NE also allows the brain to return to a state of youthful flexibility and plasticity, allowing you to learn as much as you did when you were in your youth, a time when you were exposed to many forms of stimulation.

GIVE YOURSELF A MOOD BOOST –
INCREASE NOREPINEPHRINE IN YOUR BRAIN

NE is one of your primary natural happiness chemicals. With balanced levels in your brain, your mood will be heightened, you'll experience a more positive outlook on life. Insufficient levels of norepinephrine can cause depressed moods, an inability to concentrate, an inability to cope with stress, whilst preventing short-term memories from being stored as long-term memories. In addition, NE helps regulate your sex drive. When levels are low, the sexual urge diminishes dramatically.

The power of norepinephrine to elevate mood can be easily appreciated when you look at the life of a cocaine abuser. Cocaine is so powerful that even though the abuser may have a life of desperate misery, for the few minutes whilst they ride the NE 'high' caused by its brain altering effects – they'll be in a buoyant mood. Drinking coffee also acts as a stimulant, but is much less intense. Convenience foods are all used to hit your brain with opiates. Steer clear of them.

STIMULATE NOREPINEPHRINE THE EASY WAY

Exercise significantly increases norepinephrine production, improving appetite control, mood, sex drive and mental health. Ginkgo biloba has also received a great deal of publicity recently for its NE enhancing effects. NE tends to be depleted in certain areas of the brain in Alzheimer's patients, making Ginko a valuable supplement for prevention.

Ensure you lead a busy, confident, active, yet balanced lifestyle, full of love for what you are doing and the pleasure will be there for the taking. Let's re-cap:

- ♦ NE has an arousing, sharpening effect in the brain.
- ♦ NE plays a key role in memory and learning which is why students have been known to take the drug amphetamine (also known as 'speed') to cram for exams. It has a structure similar to NE.
- ♦ Many diet pills have been taken off the market because they contained amphetamine. Excessive NE kills the appetite indirectly, causing insulin levels to drop, allowing fat to be burned as fuel. The only problem is that the body goes into a survival state ensuring that anything that is eaten gets stored away in case the artificial famine is repeated. Ultimately users gain more weight than they lost in the first place!
- ♦ Cornell researchers found that by inhibiting the synthesis of NE in rats brains, they interrupted their overall ability to remember for more than twenty-four hours.
- ♦ If you increase NE levels in your brain you'll increase your memory and learning ability as your brain returns to a youthful state of flexibility and plasticity.
- ♦ NE is also one of your primary happiness chemicals. With balanced levels in your brain, your mood will be heightened and you'll experience more energy combined with a healthier outlook on life.
- ♦ Insufficient levels of norepinephrine can cause depressed moods, an inability to concentrate, an inability to cope with stress, and prevent the storage of long-term memories.
- ♦ NE also helps regulate sex drive. If levels of NE are too low, the sexual urge diminishes dramatically.
- ♦ The raw materials necessary for the production of norepinephrine are foods high in the amino acids phenylalanine and tyrosine. Soybeans are an excellent choice.
- ♦ Exercise significantly increases norepinephrine production, improving appetite control, mood, sex life and mental health. Now for the ultimate balancing act...

4 – THE CRITICAL NEUROTRANSMITTER AXIS: DOPAMINE AND SEROTONIN

Dopamine is partly responsible for creating mental energy and alertness. As you spark the fire of your brain's dopamine neurons, your outlook on the world will become more positive, lively and buoyant. When you exercise, increased levels of dopamine will give you the edge if you need to exercise longer. If every measure isn't taken to maintain dopamine levels in your brain then serotonin is likely to take a more dominant role. These two neurotransmitters are part of a subtle balancing act.

The neurotransmitter serotonin is responsible for creating feelings of contentment and emotional control. With levels of serotonin balanced, you'll be free from the nagging temptations and cravings that plague so many people. You'll find it easy to say no to drugs, alcohol, binge eating and impulsive behaviour.

SEROTONIN: THE MASTER WEIGHT-CONTROL DRUG

If you see a chocolate bar and automatically have to have it, pay attention! You may need to balance your serotonin levels.

The substance in your brain, partly responsible for carbohydrate cravings is MCH (melanin concentrating hormone). It is made in the hypothalamus and released in the frontal lobe, a part of the brain that makes decisions about what to eat. Since serotonin is the major neurotransmitter in the frontal lobe, when MCH is released, if levels of serotonin are too low, binge eating can prevail. The only option is to naturally increase serotonin levels, and by doing so you'll avoid any cravings and have more control over your food choices. In essence, too little serotonin may mean less control over your more animal-like impulses. Whatever you do, and whatever state of mind you are in…

TAKE CONTROL AND AVOID THE PERILS OF PROZAC

Emotions and moods are affected by serotonin, a lack of which can sometimes lead to depression. Take a look at the recreational food addicts. As the market place for these foods continues to expand, more and more people are becoming addicted to foods that stimulate serotonin and insulin. The first by-product of producing excess insulin is an increase in fat storage. As serotonin levels in the brain are continually stimulated, insulin receptors wear out and the serotonin doesn't have the effect it used to have, resulting in an increase in carbohydrate craving! Gradually the downward spiral becomes so devastating, the person begins to produce more 'bad' eicosanoids and begins to suffer from depression. Is it easy to see why depression is reaching epidemic levels?

Here's where drugs like Prozac (anti-depressant drugs) come in. They are so powerful at elevating serotonin levels above normal, a bomb could explode and the user would still find it easy to remain relaxed. The downside is that the side effects rob the body of its biochemical integrity.

Prozac increases serotonin uptake in the brain, causing its users to feel an increased sense of well-being. The problem is it has potentially devastating side effects. It has been known to cause headaches, nausea, insomnia, and make its users anxious and jittery. It's also been known to cause heart seizures. A study from Harvard Medical School shows that 3.5% of the patients who took Prozac, became intensely violent and had a suicidal preoccupation after only 2-7 weeks.

If a life of disregard for your body has left you reaching for such drugs it's up to you to align yourself with the principles of RAW PERFECTION and rebalance your body. What do I mean by balance? The re-establishment of neurotransmitter equilibrium.

Consult your doctor and make the decision to leave manufactured drugs for someone else, not you! It doesn't take a genius to make the link between the number of people prescribed antidepressants who are also overweight and suffering from numerous illnesses. These drugs are fast becoming the nation's most popular mood enhancer. Too little serotonin can cause depression and violent behaviour. Too much serotonin can cause accelerated ageing, as insulin levels rise. Just like insulin and glucagon, serotonin and dopamine work in tandem. Ensure you keep the balance favourable.

THE EICOSANOID LINK BETWEEN
SEROTONIN LEVELS AND DEPRESSION

Researchers discovered in 1983 that patients suffering with depression had two to three times more 'bad' eicosanoids in their spinal fluid, compared to those with normal mental health. The bad eicosanoid they singled out the most was PGE2. They also found elevated levels of it in their saliva. By balancing eicosanoids in your favour, and increasing the good ones such as PGE1 (a mood enhancer) you gain control at a level that no drug could ever achieve!

RESTORE SEROTONIN LEVELS NATURALLY

Q: Should you devour as much carbohydrate as possible to restore serotonin levels?

A: No! Refined carbohydrates found in many convenience foods such as chocolate, crisps, breads, pastas and many snack foods are broken down quickly within your system and cause a rapid increase in blood sugar and serotonin levels. The 'high' feels good but doesn't last, leaving its victim with a nagging sense of emotional malaise. If carbohydrates are used to enhance mood, gradually they become less and less stimulating and the user needs more to induce the 'good feeling'. Talk to an obese carbohydrate addict, and they'll tell you how much they can eat in one sitting!

The excessive levels of insulin cause an over production of bad eicosanoids (such as PGE2) which are strongly associated with depression. They also destroy the sensitivity of your insulin receptors and invite obesity, increasing your chance of almost every major illness in existence. Remember that most foods high in carbohydrate are also convenience foods high in sugar and rob your body of essential nutrients.

Q: Should you consume more serotonin?
A: No. Obviously you'd increase the amount of serotonin in your brain, but too much serotonin can cause platelet aggregation, increasing your chance of a heart attack.

Q: Should you supplement your diet with the precursor of serotonin, the amino acid tryptophan?
A: No. You can't buy tryptophan over the counter because it's banned! 38 people died of an adverse reaction to a contaminated batch of the product.

Q: Should you look to eat foods that are plentiful in the amino acid tryptophan?
A: Yes, and by eating a plentiful supply of raw greens, you supply tryptophan and other amino acids necessary for optimal health. If you truly want to unwind eat almonds, chestnuts, peanuts, pecans, and walnuts and you'll feel more relaxed due to their high tryptophan content.

DOPAMINE: THE MASTER ENERGISER

Dopamine creates mental energy and alertness. The main function of dopamine is to help control physical movement. Levels of dopamine usually decrease with age, but with good dietary habits can easily be maintained.

If you see an elderly person struggle to co-ordinate a complex manoeuvre, you can assume they have low levels of dopamine in their brain. A lack of dopamine can cause a loss of co-ordination and muscular control and if the condition is left to worsen, muscular control diminishes and Parkinson's disease can often be the result.

If you are not yet convinced of the importance of maintaining your dopamine levels to ensure the serotonin-dopamine ratio is kept balanced, here are a few reasons to motivate you. High levels of dopamine:

♦ Increase your chance of achieving physical and mental longevity.
♦ Improve your overall mood and positive emotions.
♦ Increase your fat burning ability.
♦ Increase in your sex drive.
♦ Enhance your immunity.
♦ Improve your memory.
♦ Stimulate the pituitary gland to secrete growth hormone, giving you the greatest chance to burn fat, increase lean muscle mass and enhance mobility.

MANUFACTURING AND BOOSTING DOPAMINE

Dopamine and norepinephrine are manufactured in much the same way. The primary nutritional building blocks of both neurotransmitters are the amino acids tyrosine and phenylalanine.

♦ The amino acid phenylalanine boosts the functioning of your brain and also suppresses the appetite. Apricot, beansprouts, broccoli, figs, kale, peanuts, peas, potatoes, pumpkin and sesame seeds, spinach and turnip greens are all good sources.
♦ In studies where subjects were administered tyrosine, improvements were made in their ability to learn and assimilate information. Their ability to recall data improved and so did their reaction times. The tyrosine in soybeans will help you concentrate.

FEED YOUR NEUROTRANSMITTERS
AND ELIMINATE STRESS AND DEPRESSION

When you are stressed, you begin to place high demands on your nutrient reserves. The same is true of your neurotransmitters because one of the responses to stress is that your brain's neurons are fired more frequently. If this is the case, it's up to you to include enough amino acids in your diet to regenerate your neurotransmitter status. Wheatgrass juice and E3Live are abundant in amino acids. Use them! If you want to engage in another activity that naturally increases dopamine then…

GET SWEATY TOGETHER: LOVERS OF SEX REJOICE

If you feel you are a little obsessed with sex, worry no more, everything is right about sex, as long as both parties are willing! Sex stimulates dopamine. In fact, people who have active sex lives have more powerful and better functioning immune systems and are less prone to a whole host of mental disorders. Although I don't want you to think of yourself as a 'dirty rat', research shows that when male rats have orgasms, a tremendous amount of dopamine is released into the synapses in their brain. Sex is a proven method of making more dopamine, which can lead to increased longevity and a life of vigour and well-being.

DON'T BE SAD, LET NATURE LOOK AFTER YOU

People are happier in the summer because they venture outside more, and literally 'see' more sunlight. When exposed to natural sunlight the brain produces more serotonin. And for those of you in live in less temperate climates, it isn't the absence of light in the winter that prevents you from 'getting enough' of this vital nutrient, it's just you may not be going outside as much. The light is still there in the winter but the cold months prevent people from venturing outside.

Seasonal affective disorder (SAD) is caused by a lack of natural sunlight, preventing sufficient serotonin from being manufactured, causing the unfortunate carbohydrate cravings that can so often lead to a downward spiral of ill health.

The answer is to eat an abundance of chlorophyll rich foods (for liquid sunshine), exercise outside, and use mind machines to your advantage. Bright light therapy and negative ion generators will also help anyone who suffers severely with this disorder. These methods are natural, they represent the best ways in which you can increase brain serotonin levels and decrease your craving for carbohydrates.

BECOMING 'ONE' WITH NATURE

Many people suffer from lack of sleep, natural light deprivation, and the perils of convenience food? These problems cause depletion of natural serotonin levels and can be linked to a simple artificial existence.

Look at the stress that exists in society today, excessive work, redundancies, failed marriages, the problems with drugs, alcohol and smoking, not to mention the never ending supply of convenience foods, all designed to strip your pockets of money and destroy your health. Are you surprised many people feel drawn towards the so-called 'happy pills' such as Prozac? With serotonin levels decreasing, if people don't get a prescription for an antidepressant, they often try to self medicate with food. The upshot is that whilst they add extra fat to their body, they suffer the problems associated with serotonin deprivation. Your serotonin levels influence whether or not you are depressed, prone to violence, irritable, impulsive or gluttonous. Some people even consider suicide! Even though there are hundreds of neurotransmitters in your brain, serotonin may be one of the most important.

BACK TO THE ALPHA-STIM FOR ULTIMATE STIMULATION

If you are substantially overweight, you will need to rely on other measures to improve the levels of serotonin in your brain. Begin with the Alpha Stim! It is incredibly powerful and has the capacity to restore neurotransmitter equilibrium. It is at the leading edge of mind technology and can also be used as a powerful pain healing device. You'll be able to purchase one at www.lifetools.com. Let's re-cap:

- The amino acid tyrosine is the main building block of dopamine. Dopamine is linked to mental energy, vigilance, and alertness. By firing the dopamine neurons in your brain you'll become more positive, more buoyant, and even more cheerful.
- In studies where subjects were administered tyrosine, improvements were made in concentration and learning ability. Their ability to recall data improved and so did their reaction times. Soybeans are excellent sources of tyrosine, and are more effective when eaten on an empty

stomach.

♦ If you want tyrosine to enter your brain rapidly, remember that it competes with other amino acids such as tryptophan to enter your brain. Tryptophan stimulates serotonin production. So eat your tyrosine foods first.

♦ Your emotions and moods are affected by serotonin, a lack of which can often lead to depression.

♦ MCH (melanin concentrating hormone) is produced in your brain and is one factor responsible for carbohydrate craving. It is made in the hypothalamus, but is released in the frontal lobe, a part of the brain that makes decisions about what to eat. Since serotonin is the major neurotransmitter in the frontal lobe, when MCH is released, if levels of serotonin are too low, binge eating can prevail. Use mind machines to your advantage, and gain control of your neurotransmitters.

♦ One of the responses to stress is that your brain's neurons are fired more frequently. You must have enough amino acids in your diet to regenerate critical neurotransmitters.

♦ Seasonal affective disorder (SAD) is caused by a lack of natural sunlight and prevents the manufacture of serotonin. Carbohydrate cravings are at their worse during this period, but can be eliminated with chlorophyll rich foods and the use of the mind machines. Exercise (preferably outside), meditation, bright light therapy and negative ion generators are also great natural methods to combat this condition.

♦ If you want to unwind eat almonds, chestnuts, peanuts, pecans, and walnuts and you'll feel more relaxed due to their high tryptophan content.

♦ If you want to concentrate choose brazil nuts, cashews, hazelnuts, macadamias, pine nuts, and pistachios. Remember to soak and sprout all nuts!

5 – NITRIC OXIDE AND MEMORY FORMATION

In 1998 the Nobel Prize in Medicine was awarded to Robert Furchgott, Ferid Murad, and Louis Ignarro for their research into the gaseous proto-hormone known as nitric oxide. Its role in memory formation is critical. When information gets stored in your short-term memory, nitric oxide is responsible for most of the reinforcement process allowing the memory to become properly encoded in long-term memory.

If you wish to keep your brain healthy until the final moments of your life and maintain the ability to translate short-term memories into stable long-term memories then continue to ensure you eat foods that are rich in the amino acid arginine that stimulate the production of nitric oxide.

In 1958 scientists from the Soviet Union made an important discovery. They found high levels of the fat absorbing amino acid arginine present in walnuts, pine nuts, pistachios, almonds, and peanuts.

Without enough arginine in your diet, you'll find it virtually impossible to make nitric oxide. Let's re-cap:

♦ The gaseous proto-hormone known as nitric oxide is critical for reinforcing memories stored in your short-term memory allowing them to become encoded in long-term memory.
♦ Arginine also stimulates the release of growth hormone from the pituitary gland, helping to stimulate muscle growth.
♦ Arginine-rich foods include walnuts, pine nuts, pistachios, almonds, and peanuts.

THE JOY OF SEXUAL LONGEVITY

Many factors are associated with age-associated sexual decline. Poor nutrition leads to poor hormonal communication, and when testosterone levels begin to decline, libido decreases in both sexes. At approximately age 50 testosterone levels gradually decrease, causing a simultaneous drop in sexual performance. However, one hormone is never responsible for the entire picture. Take a look at how various neurotransmitters affect sexual function.

♦ Dopamine is a key element in sexual desire and its power can be easily illustrated when you look at the results of the drug L-dopa on Parkinson's patients. The drug causes a rise in dopamine and almost immediately, patients are known to experience an increase in sex drive.
♦ Acetylcholine is important in controlling the blood flow to the genitals, in males and females. It is also a key factor in the sense of relaxation that has to be present for males to achieve erections and orgasms.
♦ Norepinephrine is the neurotransmitter that must be present in adequate amounts if you want to experience sexual arousal. If you've ever complained about being too tired to have sex, you may have simply

been suffering from a norepinephrine deficit.

♦ Nitric oxide is needed for penile erections, and for enhanced blood flow to the female genitalia. As you've just discovered, the amino acid arginine is responsible for the production of Nitric oxide. Look no further than walnuts, pine nuts, pistachios, almonds, and peanuts for more arginine.

One supplement that will arouse your interest is Ginseng. For many years it has been used to enhance sexual vigour and an interesting experiment at Southern Illinois University illustrates this beautifully. Male rats given a diet that included ginseng took an average of just 14 seconds to initiate sexual contact with female rats (I like their style!), while male rats given no ginseng took an average of 100 seconds (I'm still suitably impressed – the term 'you dirty rat' begins to make perfect sense).

E3LIVE AND COMPLETE PEACE OF MIND

Your brain comprises just 2% of your total body weight, but uses an enormous 20% of your body's energy resources. If there is the slightest break in the amino acid-peptide link, you may experience memory loss, mental fatigue or nervous disorders. The amino acid peptides are precursors of the all-important neurotransmitters, which carry messages from the brain to ordinary muscles, and from the organs back to the brain. For total nourishment and complete peace of mind use E3Live daily. The complete amino acid profile of AFA within E3Live assists in nourishing the brain and nervous system.

ARE YOU READY FOR THE CHALLENGE

Recent research has shown that the mind and body have their own patterns of rest or alertness, with one predominant cycle that occurs approximately every 90 minutes, when the body stops externally oriented behaviour and takes about 15minutes to relax and replenish its energy. This is known as the ultradian rhythm. If you've ever found yourself daydreaming and feeling a little docile it was probably your body's natural stress control system kicking in.

By ignoring the relaxation response, you may develop a pattern of overriding the ultradian rhythm, often leading to burnout and disease.

Remember the salmon? Ensure you take a short break when it's time to relax and make use of the powerful mind machines! You'll feel a lot better than if you have a cup of coffee or push yourself to concentrate more.

♦ Use exercise and mind machines to stimulate your endorphins. You'll want to study more, learn more and will automatically become an information hungry machine!

♦ Use the power of raw greens and sprouted nuts and seeds to supply enough choline to produce acetylcholine.

♦ Exercise to increase the production of norepinephrine and dopamine. Also consume foods high in the amino acids tyrosine and phenylalanine. Soybeans are an excellent choice.

♦ If you want to unwind eat almonds, chestnuts, peanuts, pecans, and walnuts and you'll feel more relaxed due to their high tryptophan content, thus stimulating serotonin.

♦ If you want to concentrate choose brazil nuts, cashews, hazelnuts, macadamias, pine nuts, and pistachios. Remember to soak and sprout all nuts!

♦ Consume food high in the amino acid arginine to promote sexual vigour by stimulating nitric oxide. Look towards walnuts, pine nuts, pistachios, almonds, and peanuts for more arginine.

♦ Use Mind machines to re-establish neurotransmitter equilibrium and promote peak performance states of mind.

♦ One of the purposes of sleep is to re-establish neurotransmitter equilibrium. If you don't give your body enough building blocks to feed your neurotransmitters you'll need more sleep. AFA algae has a complete amino acid profile, delivering these building blocks.

♦ AFA found in E3Live improves children's academic performance – 1995, Sevulla et al, Univ. Centro Americana

♦ AFA found in E3Live improves Attention Deficit Disorder (ADD) – 1997 Jarratt, C, et al, The Centre for Family Wellness, Harvard, MA

♦ AFA found in E3Live reduces symptoms of Alzheimer's Disease – 1985, Cousens, Orthmedicine, Vol. 8, p.1-2

Superior nutrition specifically enhances our ability to excel as human beings – physically, mentally, emotionally and spiritually. Poor nutrition contributes to a "biologically altered brain" which functions at an inferior level. The result is increased drug addiction, alcoholism, increased hyperactivity, increased attention deficit disorders, and depression.

As you've just learned, the picture of nutritional mastery is only as good as the quality of each stroke. By learning to manipulate your neurotransmitters with the applied use of food, you've really begun to master RAW PERFECTION. It is a place where responsibility is as real as it gets. It doesn't necessarily mean you'll always be perfect, but you'll know why you feel the way you do at any given time. The aim of this chapter was to give you the key that opens the door to optimal brain function. By using the latest mind technology and the applied use of food to stimulate your brain, you'll become an information absorbing machine able to master many areas of your life.

Without energy, it's hard to achieve anything in life, but when your mind and body are working in perfect unison, anything is possible. It starts with RAW PERFECTION and as far as I'm concerned everything else is simply an extension. RAW PERFECTION makes you feel excellent. You don't need excessive amounts of money or drugs, you just need to understand the power of nutrition.

The choice is yours. A brain that waits patiently, not knowing when it's going to get it's full compliment of essential nutrients, or a brain that is powerful and on purpose.

THE RAW PERFECTION EVALUATION:
Do you eat with purpose?
Do you eat in a way that influences your mood?
Do you eat the necessary foods for the stimulation and balance of your neurotransmitters?

CHAPTER 15

INCREASING LONGEVITY AND MENTAL HEALTH THROUGH EXERCISE

Studies from the Russian space program have found that young cosmonauts subjected to the forced inactivity of space flight, fall prey to depression. However, if they are put on a schedule of regular exercise, the depression is avoided.

With this information, why do physicians often prescribe anti-depressant drugs to their depressed patients when exercise appears to be a much better prescription?! What is it about exercise that causes the reversal of depression and the re-balancing of the body? The answer lies with a class of neurochemicals called catecholamines. When physicians prescribe drugs in an effort to raise the levels of these neurochemicals, horrific side effects are often the result.

Prozac has been known to cause headaches, nausea, insomnia, and make its users anxious/jittery. It's also been known to cause heart seizures. A study from Harvard Medical School shows that 3.5% of the patients who took Prozac, became intensely violent and had a suicidal preoccupation after only 2-7 weeks.

THE ONLY SIDE EFFECT OF EXERCISE IS EUPHORIA

Exercise is holistic. By engaging in physical activity, chemical messages are sent back and forth between your brain and various muscle groups.

Part of this flow of biochemical information stimulates the production of catecholamines. Thus, whenever a doctor writes a prescription for an antidepressant, he is handing out a substitute for the body's own inner prescription, which is filled by exercise. The news that exercise offsets ageing has been well publicised, although its preventive effect on depression may not be as well known.

Exercise can also increase the production of the neurotransmitter norepinephrine and the 'feel good chemicals' endorphins – directly benefiting mood and often relieving depression. Depression is not only painful emotionally, but is destructive to memory. A number of studies have indicated that exercise is incredibly effective at dispelling depression and in many cases more effective than traditional therapies, including psychological counselling. Many problems associated with the mind and psyche can be overcome by controlling your biochemistry with correct nutrition and the application of exercise and movement.

RUN FOR YOUR LIFE!

Studies show that vigorous exercise can increase your brainpower, regardless of your current abilities. A young group of cross-country runners were tested for their overall cognitive ability during their 'off-season'. The results were recorded and compared with those taken at the end of the season. During this time they were running an average of at least thirty miles per week. By the end of the season, when tested, their cognitive ability had increased dramatically.

PLAY YOUR WAY TO GREATER INTELLIGENCE

An experiment with young, healthy monkeys also showed remarkable results. A large group was split into three:

♦ Group one was kept sedentary.
♦ Group two was given a running wheel.
♦ Group three was given an intricate series of ropes and bridges to play on.

Group two and three grew more capillaries to their brain cells and showed an increase in their cognitive abilities, allowing their brains to utilise more oxygen and nutrients. The monkeys in group three with the complex play structures grew the largest number of dendritic connections, indicating that exercise is most valuable when combined with stimulating challenges.

KEEP IT SIMPLE FOR A HIGH PERFORMANCE MIND

Even a simple exercise program of 30 minutes of walking per day over a ten-week period has been showed to be particularly effective at improving memory. One study compared the memories of a group of elderly people. Half the group were sedentary, the other half were on a walking program. Over a period of several weeks the group that exercised showed significant improvement in memory skills, while the sedentary group remained the same.

THE NATURE OF YOUTH LEADS TO NATURAL BRILLIANCE

The simplest technique for supercharging your brain is movement. The less you move, the more likely you are to suffer from cognitive decline. Think about it, in the years when your brain was developing at lightening like speed, between the moment you were born and for the first few years of your life, you engaged in all sorts of movement. When was the last time you saw a baby being rocked in a chair or in their mothers arms? They crave movement! When was the last time you saw some kids spinning around and around until they fell over? Do you remember what it was like to roll down a grassy hill? As adults we do a number of things, activities at weekends, mountaineering, sky-diving, go-carting, dancing, sports, jet ski-ing, the list goes on. All these things require movement.

HAS YOUR LIFE BECOME MOTIONLESS?

The bottom line is simple: If you've fallen into a lifestyle that demands little movement, you're more likely to suffer from motion deprivation. If you spend most of the day sitting still, whilst your fingers tap, tap, tap away on a keyboard, only to go home and slouch in front of the television, it's time you made some changes. Start now by getting up and spinning around for a few moments: Clockwise to begin with then anticlockwise.

Movement stimulates the fluids of the inner ear, known as the vestibular system. This stimulation sends a flood of electrical impulses into your cerebellum and from there into the rest of the brain, including the pleasure and learning centres of the limbic system. Motion has amazing effects on your intelligence by directly stimulating learning.

Let's dig a little deeper so you fully understand why exercise will powerfully stimulate your brainpower. You've discovered what exercise does for your body but what about your brain?

NURTURE YOUR NATURAL NERVE GROWTH FACTOR

Mary was 76 years old and lay in her hospital bed somewhere between consciousness and unconsciousness. Alzheimer's had ravaged her mind. She didn't have a wisp of a memory, or any sense of personality. Fortunately, the doctors at the Karolinska Institute in Stockholm, Sweden, believed they could help her with a bold new innovative neurological treatment. With the support of her husband, the doctors began the experimental procedure that would hopefully save her from a life of 'nothingness'.

The treatment began with the surgeons drilling a small hole into her skull and inserting a catheter directly into her brain. They then began dripping a solution containing nerve growth factor into the catheter. The goal was to stimulate Mary's neurons to grow new dendritic branches and revive enough of her neurons to bring her brain back to life. Patiently they waited. Hours turned into days, and days turned into weeks, until finally a breakthrough.

Two weeks into the treatment Mary hadn't shown any signs of improving, but after three weeks the doctors noticed something very significant. Her expressions became more lucid. As time passed, Mary became more aware of her surroundings.

The power of the treatment restored Mary's consciousness and gradually she began to speak. One day, when her husband was at her bedside, she began to talk quietly to him about their life together. Her memories came flooding back. They both cried as they held each other in their arms. Nerve growth factor saved her. It's up to you to...

STIMULATE THE WONDER DRUG NATURALLY

Nerve growth factor (NGF) is a virtual wonder drug for the brain. It is similar to a brain hormone that stimulates the regeneration of the brain: brain-derived neurotropic factor (BDNF). NGF and BDNF are both produced most abundantly when the body is physically active. In all likelihood, these important brain chemicals were created by the evolutionary process to support the brain as it withstood physical challenges.

Everyone can produce nerve growth factor on a day to day basis by doing one thing: Exercise. Physically activity maintains a youthful brain that's vital, and regenerative throughout your entire life. Exercise is the key to the fountain of youth.

The greatest effects of exercise on both NGF and BDNF are in the most plastic areas of the brain, including the hippocampus (the brain's primary memory centre). This regional concentration accounts for much of the improvement in memory experienced by people who begin to exercise. NGF and BDNF, however, also support neurons throughout the brain, in the following ways:

- ♦ They transport BDNF to the forebrain cholinergic neurons.
- ♦ They 'rescue' damaged neurons from imminent death.
- ♦ They increase the production of the important neurotransmitters, acetylcholine and dopamine, and increase the number of dopamine receptors.
- ♦ They protect brain cells by increasing the activity of neuronal free-radical scavengers.

Even though cortisol, produced by stress, destroys BDNF, exercise can help to restore levels. Exercise also helps reduce cortisol secretion by controlling insulin levels.

BURN STRESS OUT OF YOUR BODY

The more you develop your cardiovascular system, the more you develop your ability to deal with stress. When you have a low resting heart rate, as a result of exercise, it prevents your adrenal glands from overreacting to stressors, and over-secreting cortisol. Exercise increases your immunity to disease by boosting the number of 'natural killer' cells (as does E3Live), and by increasing your production of immunoglobin-A, an antibody that is one of your first lines of defence against infection.

Exercise protects your body against stress by burning off harmful stress chemicals. This is known as the tranquilliser effect and lasts for approximately four hours following exercise. It will diminish your physical response to stress dramatically during this time.

To achieve the tranquilliser effect, you must do just the right amount of exercise. In one study of joggers, those who jogged twenty-four miles per week, or about 30-45 minutes per day, experienced the tranquilliser effect the most. Those who jogged significantly less (fifteen miles per week), or significantly more (fifty-two miles per week), experienced less of the tranquilliser effect.

ENDORPHINS SWIM FREELY IN YOUR BODY AND BRAIN

Endorphins are at the heart of the tranquilliser effect. They are approximately 200 times more potent than morphine and increase approximately 500% during vigorous exercise. It only takes about fifteen to thirty minutes of exercise to stimulate their release and they remain active for about five hours – approximately the same length of time that the tranquilliser effect lasts. They are at their highest levels during the first thirty minutes after an exercise period.

In one classic study, a group of patients suffering with depression were split into three separate groups. One group was given psychotherapy for a limited number of weeks. Another group was given psychotherapy for as many weeks as the patients desired. The third group received no psychotherapy, but participated in a jogging program. At the end of the experiment, the patients in the jogging program had the lowest incidence of depression, while those in the unlimited psychotherapy program had the highest incidence.

In another study, patients suffering with depression jogged either five days a week, three days a week, or not at all. Those who jogged five days a week had significantly less depression at the end of the ten-week study. Those who jogged three days a week fared almost as well. Those who didn't jog didn't improve!

Exercise reduces depression for a number of reasons:

◆ It releases stimulating catecholamine neurotransmitters.
◆ It stimulates endorphin production.
◆ It increases oxygen flow to the brain.
◆ It helps remove neuronal debris.
◆ It stimulates the nervous system.
◆ It provides a powerful boost to self-esteem by increasing overall well-being.
◆ It improves body image and it increases feelings of personal power and responsibility.

Cognitive decline is often due to a lack of mental stimulation and a lack of physical movement. Our bodies and brains have been programmed by evolution to require physical activity.

ARE YOU READY FOR THE CHALLENGE?

I'm sure by now you've realised that exercise does more for your body and brain than you can ever imagine. Go and book a dance class, visit your local gym or maybe go for a snowboarding lesson/session! Whatever you choose to do, feel good about feeling good and remember all the reasons why exercise is going to enhance your life in every way. Here's a re-cap:

◆ Studies from the Russian space program have found that young cosmonauts subjected to the forced inactivity of space flight fall prey to depression, but when put on a schedule of regular exercise, this depression is avoided.
◆ A number of studies have indicated that exercise is incredibly effective at dispelling depression and in many cases more effective than traditional therapies, including psychological counselling.
◆ Exercise protects your body against stress by burning off harmful stress chemicals. When you have a low resting heart rate, as a result of exercise, it prevents your adrenal glands from overreacting to stressors, and over-secreting cortisol. In fact, approximately four hours following exercise, people experience a tranquilliser effect that diminishes their physical response to stress. Remnants of the tranquilliser effect may remain for up to twenty-four hours.
◆ Endorphins, which are 200 times more potent than morphine, increase approximately 500% during vigorous exercise. After they are released,

they remain active for about five hours – approximately the same length of time that the tranquilliser effect lasts.

♦ A group of cross-country runners were tested for cognitive ability during their off season, and again at the end of the season. They scored significantly higher after running at least thirty miles per week.

♦ Even a simple exercise program of 30 minutes walking per day over a ten-week period has been showed to be particularly effective at improving memory.

♦ Exercise is essential for optimal brain function. It supplies the brain with nerve growth factor, it reduces stress and it enhances neuronal metabolism.

♦ Nerve growth factor (NGF) is a virtual wonder drug for the brain. It is similar to a brain hormone that also stimulates regeneration of the brain: brain-derived neurotropic factor (BDNF). NGF and BDNF are both produced most abundantly when the body is physically active.

♦ Exercise increases your immunity to disease by boosting your immune system's number of 'natural killer' cells, and by increasing your production of immunoglobin-A, an antibody that is one of your first lines of defence against infection.

So there you have it, exercise increases the brain's uptake of oxygen and glucose. It speeds the removal of necrotic debris from brain cells. It enhances the production of various neurotransmitters such as norepinephrine and dopamine, and increases the availability of brain-related enzymes, such as Co-enzyme Q-10. It increases the output of endorphins. It decreases cortisol output leading to less perceived stress in any situation. It has a tranquillising effect on the brain decreasing any chance of depression. It helps lower blood pressure by helping to control insulin levels. And it helps stabilise blood sugar levels (thereby helping to stabilise mood and energy) again by assisting in the control of insulin. Exercise also burns calories, increases muscle mass, and strengthens bones. So the question becomes, can you be bothered? If your answer isn't a resounding YES, read this chapter until it is!

THE RAW PERFECTION EVALUATION:
Are you using exercise to enhance your mind as well as your body?

EMBRⓘⓘⓘⓘⓘⓘ

PART FOUR

EMBRACING AN UNLIMITED FUTURE

CHAPTER 16

MAXIMISE YOUR LIFE-SPAN:
THE TRUE NATURE OF RAW PERFECTION

If someone offered you a magical pill that could guarantee all the above and more, would you say, "No thanks, I'd prefer to die from some crippling disease." The answer is obvious!

Even though most people would choose to avoid a crippling disease, you still hear the common catchphrase, "I don't want to live a long life, who wants to live for a long time if they are going to be senile and need looking after?" Or, "Everybody dies of something, sooner or later, so you might as well die from something that makes you feel good." But just stop for a minute. If you think that being alive for a shorter period of time will mean you'll remain mobile and fully functional until you pass away – Think again. Whether you die at 55 or 155, one thing is for certain, you are more likely to die from a disabling illness early on in life than in later life.

If you have the genetic potential to live between 120 and 140 years of age, there can only be one conclusion. To die any earlier means you must have engaged in daily habits or rituals that accelerated the ageing process, causing you to die prematurely.

Take a look at the suffering endured by victims of cancer, crippling strokes, or Alzheimer's disease. These horrific scenes cause people to see sense, not stupidity. What is my point? As usual it's simple. If you don't concern yourself with taking care of things now, you'll never reach your genetic potential. If you don't reach your genetic potential then the likelihood of you dying from a killer disease increases dramatically. It's better to die later than sooner, in peace, not in pain. And it's better to die as yourself, rather than a poor, brain-destroyed victim of Alzheimer's.

It's up to you to see the world the way it is and then make it the way you want it. Use the principles to make your life as perfect as possible and prepare to remain youthful in a world that seems to age faster than necessary.

REACHING OUT FOR THE MAXIMUM

When I found out that the likely maximum lifespan of a human being is in the region of 120 to 150 years (or above), I was curious to say the least. I wanted to know everything that could allow me to reach this maximum. Out of a range of possibilities, there does exist a magic formula that dramatically lengthens the life span in animals. This magic formula is likely to work for humans because it's been tested on almost every species alive to date. If you want to reach your genetic potential and live a totally vivacious life, it's time you learnt about …

THE GREAT CALORIE RESTRICTION EXPERIMENTS

University of California expert on ageing, Dr. Roy Walford, has reported that cutting down on food consumption is the only method that retards the ageing process, extending the maximum life-span of warm-blooded animals. You may be thinking that you are too old to begin applying this principle, but animal studies indicate a possible 10-20% increase in life span by reducing calories, starting as late as middle age. Even though experts use the terms 'calorie restriction', 'underfeeding', or even 'under nutrition' I prefer to use another term that is more in line with the principles of RAW PERFECTION. The term I use is 'An Optimal Minimum'.

The definition for 'An Optimal Minimum' is eating as much of every nutrient your body needs, but no more or no less. The problem with the dietary habits of western civilisation is that they are built around high calorie, nutrient deficient foods that lack any real 'life-force'. With an optimum minimum, calories are restricted, but not at the expense of vital nutrients or high vibrational raw foods.

Calorie restriction promotes longevity by providing a number of physiological advantages.

♦ It places less strain on the organs of digestion and assimilation.
♦ It produces fewer free radicals.
♦ It boosts levels of antioxidant enzymes by as much as 400%.
♦ It increases immune system strength by up to 300%.
♦ It lowers blood insulin levels and cholesterol.
♦ It increases glucose tolerance and lowers blood pressure.

For example, studies have shown that 'optimum minimum' eating has achieved a remarkable 300% life-extension with fish and a 60% increase in lifespan with rats. Rhesus monkeys on a calorie-restricted diet have leaner bodies, lower blood pressure, more optimal cholesterol levels, lower blood glucose and lower fasting insulin than the same animals, fed a higher level of calories. Communication between hormones is also enhanced due to less waste build-up, in and around cells.

Melatonin and DHEA normally decrease during ageing but begin to rise when calorie restriction/optimal minimum eating prevails.

BECOMING OLDER AND WISER
IN A WORLD OF MENTAL DETERIORATION

Dr Walford also indicated that as well as maximising lifespan, calorie restriction can prevent the brain from deteriorating. His experiments indicate that caloric restriction prevents the decline of the dopamine receptors in the brain cells of animals. If this can be carried over to humans, it would mean that the action of one of the most important neurotransmitters could be enhanced. It isn't unusual for dopamine to decline in the elderly, causing restricted bodily movement, including Parkinson's disease.

Another one of Dr. Walford's experiments indicated that the function of the dendrites within brain cells is also improved when calories are restricted. Again, if this applied to humans, it would be a major breakthrough in longevity. The ability to grow new dendrites is one of the most important aspects of brain plasticity. In recent years, researchers have found that new dendritic connections can be forged up until the very last moments of life, allowing your brain to regenerate as long as you're alive. Anything that might stimulate this regeneration is obviously valuable, but remember that...

THERE ALWAYS EXISTS A BARE MINIMUM

Although this may come as no surprise, there is one thing you must remember once you've decided to restrict the calories in your diet. No matter how much you restrict your calorie intake, you must ensure you consume adequate amounts of raw greens, such as E3Live/wheatgrass juice, to meet your daily requirement of essential amino acids. You must also consume adequate amounts of raw plant fats to meet your daily requirement of essential fatty acids, and ensure you get your carbohydrates from raw foods such as fruits, vegetables and sprouted nuts, seeds, beans, and lentils. By eating raw foods you'll include an abundance of micronutrients from vitamins and minerals to phytochemicals, enzymes and antioxidants. Your colon must also be clean to allow the maximum absorption of nutrients. Have you had a series of colonics yet?

CUT CALORIES BY 40%
AND WATCH YOUR BODY RETURN TO YOUTH

As long as you utilise every other principle in this book, if you eat an 'optimal minimum' and cut your calorie intake by 40%, you can expect to increase your maximum life span, the functionality of your neurotransmitter receptors, your learning ability, your immune system function, your kidney function and the length of female fertility.

You can also expect to decrease your body fat percentage, your loss of bone mass, your blood glucose levels, your insulin levels, your chance of cancer, your chance of autoimmune disease, your blood lipid levels, your chance of heart disease and your chance of diabetes.

PUT THE SHOVEL DOWN AND STOP FILLING YOUR FACE!

There are many ways to look at why calorie restriction works, maybe it's not that calorie restriction actually provides these benefits, but that gluttony promotes the decrease in longevity. When you look around and see what most people shovel into their bodies, is it any wonder many people die so prematurely? The body can only handle so much waste before it weakens and breaks down.

Dietary restriction experiments in animals have been going on for at least 60 years. Everything from primitive single-cell pond animals to small mammals (such as rats and mice) have been successfully tested on. Just imagine what happens when you combine all these principles together...

SAVE THE ELDERLY FROM AN EARLY GRAVE

In the 1960s, a team of scientists in Spain reported an experiment with two groups of elderly people in a nursing home. One group ate their usual diet, whilst the next group restricted their calorie intake whilst increasing their intake of nutrients. After three years, the second group had experienced 50% less illness and half the rate of death compared to the first.

THE THREE PIVOTAL POINTS
OF 'OPTIMAL MINIMUM' EATING

By eating an 'optimal minimum' you can slow ageing right down and produce amazing results. Here are three very powerful reasons why:

PIVOTAL POINT NO. 1 – By overexposing yourself to free radical attack, you simply accelerate the ageing process. One of the easiest ways to do this is to eat too many calories.

According to Dr. Lawrence E. Lamb, M.D., "The repair of cell membranes in animals on restricted caloric intake even suggests the possibility that calorie limitation could help reverse earlier changes caused by oxidants."

Longevity, or the risk of mortality, correlates very well with blood levels, or dietary intakes of vitamin C, vitamin E, vitamin A and beta-carotene. A recent study published in the American Journal of Clinical Nutrition followed 11,178 people between the ages of 67 and 105 over ten years. The overall risk of death was reduced by 42% for those who took supplements of both vitamins C and E.

PIVOTAL POINT NO.2 – 'Optimum minimum' eating increases the production of protective enzymes. These are as follows:

1. Superoxide dimutase (SOD), known to reduce the superoxide free radicals to hydrogen peroxide.
2. Glutathione peroxidase, known to reduce hydrogen peroxide to water.
3. Glutathione catalase, known to also reduce hydrogen peroxide to water.

By eating an 'optimum minimum' you also increase your production of melatonin, another efficient scavenger of hydroxyl free radicals, the true villains that promote cellular damage.

Do you remember what you learned about wheatgrass juice in chapter 2? Wheatgrass is a superior food source of a Superoxide dimutase (SOD). Laboratory trials and clinical tests have proven SOD is a safe and effective enzyme that protects us from cell damage. Most cellular damage is caused by superoxides, infection, ageing, radiation, and poisoning by bad food, air, or drugs. Wheatgrass juice, along with E3Live should be the first thing you drink in the morning, and the last thing you think of at night. It costs next to nothing and is more powerful than every nutritional supplement in existence.

PIVOTAL POINT NO. 3 – Reduce calories by eating an 'optimum minimum' and you take the most important step towards slowing the ageing process. When you reduce calories you reduce insulin production, promoting a more favourable balance between itself and glucagon, whilst encouraging a more favourable eicosanoid balance, optimising hormonal communication throughout your body.

When you reduce insulin secretion, you automatically stabilise blood glucose levels and minimise the stimulation of cortisol. Excess cortisol inhibits the formation of eicosanoids and kills cortisol-sensitive cells in the brain and the thymus. An example of a community that abide by these principles are the...

THE HUNZAS, A COMMUNITY OF CENTENARIANS

Let me introduce you to the Hunzas, a community that live in the Mountain Peaks of the Himalayas, where the borders of Kashmir, China, India and Afghanistan converge. They have a population of only 30,000, but a reputation that has been spread far and wide around the world. They have an amazing record of producing centenarians, many living up to ages of 145 years.

If you were to visit them you'd realise they know nothing of disease and are endowed with remarkably high levels of health and vibrancy. I bet you never even realised that there is a community on this planet where cancer and heart disease is unheard of. What about arthritis, varicose veins, constipation, stomach ulcers or appendicitis? No chance! Even mumps, measles and chicken pox are unheard of. So before I share with you some secrets of this amazing community. Take a look at the reputation of the Hunzas:

◆ The Hunzas possess boundless energy/enthusiasm and are very serene.
◆ At one hundred years old, a Hunza is considered neither old nor elderly.
◆ They consider physical and intellectual maturity to be at its highest when they've been alive for 100 years.
◆ It is not uncommon for Hunza men to father children at the age of 80.
◆ Hunza women at the age of 80 look no different from the most youthfully slim and vibrant 40-year-olds we see in our society. Hunza women remain slim, supple and graceful, and maintain excellent posture.
◆ The Hunzas have no idea what it means to be obese. Cellulite is unknown to them.
◆ Hunza men have been seen carrying what we'd consider backbreaking loads, up steep mountain paths, at the age of 100.

Their first belief is simple: The food you eat is your best medicine, and a study conducted by Dr. MacCarrisson can only confirm this basic law. The experiment involved using 3 groups of mice, each eating a different diet.

1. The first group, nourished exclusively on Hunza food, flourished and enjoyed spectacular health.
2. The second group was fed a diet similar to that of the people of neighbouring Kashmir. They developed a number of diseases.
3. The third group received a typical British diet, and quickly developed all the symptoms of neurathenia (nervous weakness, exhaustion and irritability).

IF YOU ARE WAITING FOR THE SECRET, IT CAN BE SUMMED UP IN ONE WORD: FRUGALITY

They eat only two meals a day. They rise at 5a.m. but don't eat their first meal until 12 noon. Hunza food is completely natural, containing no chemical additives and by eating small portions, they show a high degree of vitality and enthusiasm. Their preferred fruits and vegetables include potatoes, string beans, peas, carrots, turnip, squash, spinach, lettuce, apples, pears, peaches, apricots, cherries and blackberries. They eat many nuts such as walnuts, hazelnuts, almonds, beechnuts etc. Nuts often constitute an entire meal or are eaten with fruit, or mixed into salad. Almonds are eaten whole, or used to make oil through a process that has been passed from generation to generation. When they do eat meat, which is quiet rare, small portions are eaten, chicken being their most common source.

Much of the water the Hunzas drink comes from glaciers, and carries colloidal minerals. A high raw diet in alignment with the principles of RAW PERFECTION will supply an abundance of colloidal minerals.

SURVIVING THE WINTER WITH SPROUT POWER

In his book Healthy Hunzas, John Tobe reports that the Hunzas use the power of sprouts to survive the long, cold winters, in the Himalayan mountains. Sprouts provide them with vital nutrients, and when winter turns to spring and food supplies are low, the Hunzas rely on sprouts as a source of vitamins, enzymes, and energy.

HARNESSING THE PRINCIPLES OF THE HUNZAS

In addition to daily physical exercise, the Hunzas practice certain basic yoga techniques, notably yogic breathing. Yogic breathing is very slow, deep and rhythmic, and makes use of the entire thoracic cavity.

Relaxation is the key to health and the Hunzas, both young and old, practice it regularly. You can do the same and spread 'powernaps' throughout your day. I tend to use short 10-minute sessions on my Proteus light/sound machine and generally get amazing results. Many mind machines can train you to reach deep states of relaxation very quickly.

Rather than work in quick bursts, the Hunzas know they can work much longer if they are not tense and take regular breaks. They enter a state of deep relaxation and focus inwards, listening to the silence of their soul. Another way to rejuvenate your body and mind is to take twenty deep, long, slow breaths.

THE HUNZAS MAINTAIN A POWERFUL MIND

One thing that has been proven by modern medicine is that when the mind becomes dull – due to a lack of curiosity or interest, it begins to deteriorate, and when the mind deteriorates, the body does as well, resulting in muscular, cellular and circulatory degeneration. The difference with the Hunzas is that they rejoice at the thought of getting old because to them, age equals wisdom and maturity. When they are older they are a greater value to society.

Hunzas prefer to remain physically active for as long as possible. They follow the principle that 'to live' means 'to move'. If you want to adopt the mindset of a Hunza start by thinking that your youth (the first stage in life), ends at around 50, next comes the middle years, which last until 80 and finally comes the age of plenitude, the best years of your life!

Hunza people live everyday as if their whole life were ahead of them. In some respects they are like children – happy in the present moment, not worried about the future.

ARE YOU USING THE POWER OF WILD GREENS
TO MAXIMISE YOUR POTENTIAL?
THE DAGASTANIS ARE...

In the Caucasus Mountains of southern Russia, and on the coast of the Caspian Sea, live the inhabitants of the Dagestan republic. Out of the 2million residents of this province, the oldest recorded Dagestani lived to a ripe old age of 146, with many reaching ages between 120-130 years. Their diet consists of a plethora of wild grasses and weeds. Chickweed, shepherd's purse, rose hips, camomile, lambs quarters, thistle, thyme, sorrel, yellow dock, vetch, daisy, clover, wild marjoram, oregano, amaranth, mustard, garlic, and the grasses of wheat, barley, and oats make up the mainstay of their diet. With the young leaves they create mouth-watering salads and with the older more fibrous ones they create health-giving soups and stews. Even seeds are used to make tea, breads and pancakes after being crushed into a powder.

Intrigued at their amazing health, researchers from the Caspian medical college examined 154 alpine residents. 130 lived at altitudes of 6400 ft above sea level, whilst 24 lived on flat lands. The age range of the group was between 85 and 116 years and in an effort to learn the secrets of this group, the researchers moved into their homes for 10-12 days. They bombarded them with questions, and tests, weighing them, whilst examining their dietary/lifestyle habits.

Those who seem to be maximising their longevity have the most consistent habits. They start their day by waking between 5am and 6am and rather than eat a 'hearty' breakfast, they drink nothing but tea made from weeds and grasses. This tea is also drunk before and after meals for increasing appetite and improving digestion. Then between 9am and 10am they eat a light breakfast. The 90-year-olds ate the most green 'chlorophyll' rich foods, but even the children included these health-giving foods in their diet.

DEAD NUTRITIONISTS LEAD BY EXAMPLE!

In their quest for the secret of eternal youth, many nutritionists have written books on the subject of longevity, certain in their assumption of what constitutes perfect health. Those who are old may give you valuable tips. Those who are dead, lead by example! Nathan Pritikin, Professor Arnold Ehret and Dr Norman Walker all have two things in common. Firstly they are dead! Secondly they all wrote nutritional books claiming they could lead you down the path to health and longevity. So, who lived the longest? Let's take a look.

The Pritikin Program for Diet and Exercise, was a popular book during the 1970s. Nathan Pritikin popularised a diet that consisted of mostly complex carbohydrates and minimal cholesterol, fat and protein. He died of leukaemia at the pinnacle of his success at age 69, from the complications surrounding an experimental medical treatment.

Ehret had a different focus. He specialised in long fasts and a diet rich in fruit and green leafy vegetables. Everyone thought he was in exceptional health. Unfortunately he focused more on fruit than fresh raw greens and in 1922 at age 56 he died from a fractured skull after falling backwards and hitting his head! Can you imagine what the condition of his bones must have been like! This is a warning! Ensure you don't dissolve your bones away by not eating enough calcium rich raw foods – skull fractures very rarely cause death!

Norman Walker was famous in the USA for his electrical juicers. Not only did he advise eating a diet high in fruit and vegetables, but he also recommended a variety of juice cocktails. One of my favourite books, 'Colon health', written by Norman Walker highlights the importance of having a series of regular colonics. This man was a genius! His remarkable recovery from a so-called 'terminal illness' in his thirties gave him a great foundation of health on which to build. The foundation must have been strong as he lived to 109! He was vital and alive up until the morning of his death, where he was found dead in his study.

Whether you call it common sense, need scientific proof, or need a first hand example of a dead raw foodist – raw foodism is the only way to truly succeed. When raw greens, raw plant fats, fruits, sprouts, salads and vegetables are correctly used and understood exceptional health is the result. In chapter 2 you discovered the power of greens, and I hope that message has remained strong throughout this book. No vegetarian, vegan or raw food lifestyle is complete without them. Even a cooked food eater can benefit massively from such advice. Vegetables supply nutrients in concentrations not found in fruit, especially calcium. Take Norman Walker's example to heart, and become an example yourself! 750g of greens per day, juiced, blended or eaten raw will help guarantee strong bones and scintillating health!

ARE YOU READY FOR THE CHALLENGE?

Your training is nearly complete, and the RAW PERFECTION 'black belt' is just around the corner, but remember, like any martial art, the black belt is only the beginning. With an abundance of energy and enthusiasm for life, you can achieve anything you desire. The only question is: Where have you set the limits? The same is true of this chapter. You have the potential to live pain free and full of vitality well into your hundreds and beyond! Use what you know and the gateway to success will open itself very wide. Here's a re-cap that'll remind you why 'optimal minimum' eating is the ultimate goal:

♦ If you have the potential to live between 120 and 140 years old there can only be one conclusion. To die any earlier means you must have engaged in daily habits or rituals that over time caused you to accelerate the ageing process. Do you want to suffer with cancer, be crippled by a stroke, or ravaged by Alzheimer's?

♦ University of California expert on ageing, Dr. Roy Walford, has reported that calorie restriction is the only method that retards ageing and extends the maximum life span of warm-blooded animals. Animal studies indicate a possible 10-20% increase in life span by cutting down on calories, starting as late as middle age.

♦ Calorie restriction promotes longevity by providing a number of physiological advantages: It places less strain on the organs of digestion and assimilation, it produces fewer free radicals, it boosts levels of antioxidant enzymes by as much as 400%, it increases immune system strength by up to 300% and most importantly of all, lowers blood insulin levels.

♦ Studies with fish have achieved a remarkable 300% increase in life-extension. Studies with rats have produced a 60% increase in life-extension. Rhesus monkeys on a calorie-restricted diet have leaner bodies and lower blood pressure, cholesterol, blood glucose and fasting insulin (see next chapter for explanation) than the same animals fed a higher level of calories.

♦ Melatonin and DHEA normally decrease during ageing but begin to rise with calorie restriction.

♦ Dr Walford indicated that calorie restriction could prevent your brain from deteriorating during the ageing process. Caloric restriction prevents the decline of the dopamine receptors in the brain cells of animals, enhancing one of the most important neurotransmitters.

♦ Another one of Dr. Walford's experiments indicated that the function of dendrites within the brain cells also improved by restricting calories in animals.

♦ If you eat an 'optimal minimum' and cut your calorie intake by 40%, you can expect to increase your maximum life span, the functionality of your neurotransmitter receptors, your learning ability, your immune system function, your kidney function and the length of your female fertility. You can also expect to decrease your body fat percentage, your loss of bone mass, your blood glucose levels, your insulin levels, your chance of cancer, your chance of autoimmune disease, your blood lipid levels, your chance of heart disease and your chance of diabetes.

♦ 'Optimum minimum' eating increases the production of superoxide dimutase, glutathione peroxidase and glutathione catalase – three very powerful protective enzymes.

♦ By using the principle of 'optimal minimum' eating, you can begin to think like a Hunza. Their perception of life is as follows: The first stage of life, called the age of youth, ends at around 50, next comes the middle years, which last until 80 and finally comes the age of plenitude, the best years of their life!

♦ Healthy ageing is having a good quality of life and quantity of life. The ideal is to die as young as possible as late as possible.

♦ Over a 40-year period, if you sleep one hour less per day, you gain 15 extra days each year, totalling 1.7 years over the course of 40 years. In that time you could master anything. Think about it!

The concept of treating food as if it were a drug began some 2500 years ago when Hippocrates said, "Let food be your medicine, and let medicine by your food."

THE RAW PERFECTION EVALUATION:
Are you extending your life by *happily* eating an 'optimal minimum'?
Have you mastered each principle enough to utilise these fine distinctions?

You may have lost unwanted body fat, increased your lean body mass, enhanced every aspect of your mental health, and feel superior in every way, but don't let your progress stop there! To highlight the power of RAW PERFECTION endeavour to find out what changes have taken place at the cellular level.

CHAPTER 17

THE PARAMETERS OF SUCCESS:
DON'T JUST BE AFFECTED BY THE PLACEBO EFFECT, GET EVERY PARAMETER CHECKED

Apart from the way you feel on a day to day basis, the only way to judge the success of RAW PERFECTION is to have your doctor test a variety of parameters within your body. The easiest one is the litmus test where you can check the acid/alkaline balance of your body. Simply visit your nearest chemist and pick up some blue litmus paper and swipe it through your midstream urine. If the paper turns red or pink it is likely you've been engaging in too many acid forming habits. If it stays blue or violet then your body is maintaining a more favourable slightly alkaline state. The litmus test is a great way to get feedback over your current habits, but shouldn't be used to evaluate long-term health. Another excellent test is to have your blood pressure measured. Blood pressure is very sensitive to hyperinsulinemia. An average reading is around 120/80mm Hg and anything around 160/100mm Hg can be cause for concern. A more thorough method of testing is to obtain results from the following tests.

Test	Ideal Ranges
Fasting tryglycerides	Fasting tryglycerides should be under 100 mg/dl
HDL cholesterol	HDL cholesterol should be more than 50mg/dl
Fasting-triglyceride to HDL cholesterol ratio	The ratio should be less than 2.0
Glycosylated haemoglobin (HgA1C)	HgA1C should be less than 5%
Fasting insulin	less then 10 μU units/ml
Percentage body fat:	
Males	Less than 15%
females	Less than 22%

If you want to prove that the principles of RAW PERFECTION are second to none, get tested by your local GP and get tested often, every three months to begin with.

FASTING INSULIN – Although a great starting point, this is a very expensive test and requires careful sample preparation to ensure accurate results. The great thing about this test is it will tell you how high your insulin levels are. Elevated insulin levels of Type 2 diabetic patients are strongly correlated with an increased chance of heart disease, stroke, obesity, blindness, kidney failure, amputation and impotence. The New England Journal of Medicine, in 1996, showed that even the slightest elevations in fasting insulin levels made it easier to predict who would or would not develop heart disease.

GLYCOSYLATED HAEMOGLOBIN LEVELS – Another relatively expensive test and yet very simple. The results will indicate how well you've been keeping your blood sugar levels controlled on a long-term basis. It will also highlight the amount of cortisol your body is producing. With a greater control of your blood sugar levels cortisol will be minimised. The glycosylated haemoglobin in Type 2 diabetics is between 8% and 11%. One aim of diabetic patients is to get their glycosylated haemoglobin under 7%. If they manage to do this they can almost expect to be free from the long-term complications associated with diabetes.

THE RATIO OF FASTING TRYGLYCERIDES TO HDL CHOLESTEROL – This is an easily accessible blood test. The higher the ratio, the higher your insulin levels. If you want to slow down (if not reverse) the ageing process, then lower your ratio of fasting triglycerides:HDL cholesterol. The ratio should be below 2, and ideally less than 1. If the ratio is greater than 4, you are ageing faster than normal. In virtually all Type 2 diabetics studied, the ratio is always greater than four.

Research from Harvard Medical School produced a report demonstrating that the ratio of tryglycerides to HDL cholesterol is a powerful predictor of heart disease. They compared individuals who'd recently survived a first heart attack with controls of a similar age, weight and background. Those with the highest ratios were found to have 1600% increased likelihood of a heart attack than those who had lower ratios. Smoking causes a 400% increased chance of a heart attack, whilst high cholesterol increases the likelihood by 200%. Lower your fasting tryglyceride to HDL cholesterol ratio and you'll increase your chances of a longer, healthier life.

The famous Lifestyle Heart Trial that ended in 1995 also confirms the dangers of low-fat, high carbohydrate eating. In this trial, cardiovascular patients with high triglycerides:HDL cholesterol ratios engaged in stress reduction techniques, exercise and low-fat, high carbohydrate/vegetarian eating habits for five years. The only parameter reported was the triglyceride:HDL cholesterol ratio, an excellent indicator of insulin levels.

The average triglyceride:HDL cholesterol ratio was very high at the beginning of the trial at 5.7 but, after five years engaging in this program, the average had increased to 7.1. If you thought this way of life was healthy, take a look at what the lead author of that study, Dr K. Lance Gould, (a respected cardiologist in the U.S.) had to say in 1996, in a letter sent to the Journal of the American Medical Association:

'Frequently, triglyceride levels increase and HDL-cholesterol levels decrease for individuals on vegetarian, high carbohydrate diets. Since low HDL-cholesterol, particularly with high triglycerides incurs substantial risk of coronary events, I do not recommend a high-carbohydrate strict vegetarian diet.'

I wonder what would happen if the mainstay of the vegetarian diet was greens and green juices such as wheatgrass juice, raw plant fats, and fibrous fruits, vegetables and sprouts. Most vegetarian diets consist of pasta, potatoes, rice, cheese and sauces loaded with sugar.

YOUR BODY FAT PERCENTAGE - Forget your weight! Think in terms of your body fat percentage. Your body fat percentage is related directly to the level of insulin in your body. If your body fat percentage is high, you are likely to be ageing faster than normal.

THE BRUTAL TRUTH IS ONLY A BLOOD TEST AWAY

Your blood represents the brutal truth about your health. It can't lie, it can't deceive and it can't misinform. I believe the further you are away from RAW PERFECTION, the closer you are towards chronic disease and accelerated ageing! If the following values apply to you then you are hyperinsulinemic, ageing faster than normal and putting your health at risk.

♦ Your tryglycerides are greater than 200mg/dL.
♦ Your HDL cholesterol less than 35mg/dL.
♦ Your fasting insulin greater than 15 units/ml.
♦ Your glycosylated haemoglobin greater than 9 %.
♦ Your fasting-triglyceride:HDL cholesterol ratio is greater than 4.

ACCELERATED AGEING LEADS TO ACCELERATED DEATH: TAKE YOUR FOOT OFF THE INSULIN ACCELERATOR AND SLOW DOWN THE AGEING PROCESS

As you age, various biological markers of ageing change within your body as you get closer to your last day on earth. Take a look at what happens to the biological markers as you age:

♦ Insulin resistance increases.
♦ Systolic Blood Pressure increases.
♦ Percentage body fat and lipid ratios increase.
♦ Glucose tolerance decreases.
♦ Aerobic capacity decreases.
♦ Muscle mass and strength decreases.

♦ Temperature regulation decreases in efficiency.
♦ Immune function diminishes.

The list of physiological changes can all be related to excessive levels of
the hormone insulin! Take your foot off the ageing accelerator by eating
foods that maintain optimal hormonal control. The more you focus on
the habits of success the easier you'll find it to remain in control.

THE MYSTERY OF AWARENESS UNCOVERED

Isn't it amazing that in two years, 98% of the atoms in your body will
have been exchanged for new ones? It may sound absurd, but 24 months
from now you could have totally rebuilt your body.

Ageing is a natural process, but it's worth noting that there are
some organisms that never age, such as single-celled amoebas, algae,
and protozoa. Parts of you also remain ageless – your emotions, ego,
personality type, IQ, and other mental characteristics, as well as vast
portions of your DNA. Physically, it makes no sense to say that the
water and minerals in your body are ageing, for what is 'old water' or
'old salt'? These components alone make up 70% of your body. The
honeybee at certain times of the year can shift its hormones and
completely reverse its age. In the human body, shifts in hormones may
not be as dramatic, but there is enough latitude that on any given day,
your hormone profile may be younger than the day, month, or even year
before. The last place you can exert influence over your age is in your
mind…

SHIFT YOUR MENTAL STATE AND ADD YEARS TO YOUR LIFE

When someone shifts their awareness they can have a dramatic effect on
their own physiology. It's as simple as placing your attention on
memories that you really enjoyed, past triumphs or exciting times in
your life. When you think about your first love, you trigger a cascade of
hormones associated to that experience. If you consistently focus on a
time when you succeeded at something you'll continually feel the
emotion of success and your whole biochemistry will confirm this.

TURNING BACK THE HANDS OF TIME

To illustrate this principle, a psychologist, Ellen Langer and her colleagues at Harvard conducted an experiment in 1979 in an effort to reverse the biological age of a group of men. The men in the group were all over 75 years of age and in good health. Her theory was that by manipulating their environment, she could get them to experience life as it was twenty years ago.

They met at a country resort for 1 week, knowing they'd be subject to innumerable tests both physically and mentally. Each one came alone, with no reminders of any year past 1959, no newspapers, photos, tapes or CDs, or anything that would take their focus off of 1959.

At the resort, every last effort was made to ensure their life would be similar to the one they lived 20 years ago. Whenever they picked up a paper or magazine, it would be from the year 1959. The music played was from 1959. Every piece of furniture was from 1959. In fact, every last little trinket was from 1959. One of the rules of the week was that the men had to fully associate to the experience of being in the year 1959. Every conversation, movement, gesture, catchphrase, thought and feeling had to be related to their life in 1959 and to make this easier the entire environment was set up as if they'd gone back in time. ID photos were given to each subject, with pictures taken from 1959. They referred to all current affairs as if it was 1959 and talked about their jobs as if they were still in employment.

Langer and her team used this time to measure each and every marker of biological age. They measured physical strength, posture, perception, cognition, and short-term memory, along with thresholds of hearing, sight, and taste.

The experiment by the Harvard team gave each man a chance to alter his self-image, hypothesising that the shift in self-awareness would directly influence the ageing process.

Whether you call it play-acting or not, the results were remarkable! Everything about their life improved. Their memories became sharper, their manual dexterity improved, their mobility improved and they became more self-sufficient. They cooked their own meals, cleaned up after themselves and totally adopted the role of a 55-year-old. One week produced the following results:

♦ Their faces looked younger by an average of three years.
♦ Their fingers lengthened (fingers usually shorten with age).

♦ Their joints regained flexibility.
♦ Their posture straightened out.
♦ Their muscle strength increased.
♦ Their hearing sense and vision improved remarkably.
♦ Their intelligence increased.

Although a landmark in the study of ageing, Professor Langer attributed the success of the study to three factors:

1. The group behaved as if they were younger. Could you also do this?
2. They were treated like 55 year olds, rather than 75 year olds (like at home).
3. They had to follow complex procedures as part of their daily routine. Could you also increase your level of stimulation? Maybe you could start playing a musical instrument, or rekindle your enjoyment of art, such as painting. Maybe you could engage in various sports endeavours or even just begin to challenge your mind with crossword puzzles? The options are endless.

THE REMARKABLE RESULTS OF TIME TRAVEL

By becoming inner time travellers, Langer was able to create an environment that allowed the men to travel back in time by 20 years. The most exciting result was that their whole physiology followed. Stop for a minute now and consider all the ways you could creatively manipulate your mind to allow these changes to occur. Remember the more vivid your participation, the closer you will come to duplicating the body chemistry of youth.

Stimulate your mind today and re-access old pathways of youth, making them new again, and again, until you feel the energy radiate and reverberate throughout your entire body and out into the world. It's up to you to change your inner experience and travel back in time using the biochemistry of memory as your vehicle.

VISUALISATION:
ANOTHER VEHICLE TO ENHANCE HEALTH

There's now scientific proof that visualisation works. Researchers using high tech equipment have shown that when you 'see' pictures, or 'hear' music in your mind, parts of your brain are stimulated and send messages to your endocrine and nervous system. Mental imagery actually triggers physical responses in your body.

Your imagination is very powerful. Have you ever been lying in bed at night and thought you heard a door open downstairs? Did your heart start pounding as you broke out into a sweat, wondering whether there was an intruder or not? If there was an intruder, I apologise for bringing the memory to the forefront of your mind. But if there wasn't an intruder, you can see how the threat was all in your imagination.

In the 1970s, Dr Carl Simonton, a cancer specialist at the University of Oregon, conducted a study in which he found that 30 out of 159 terminal cancer patients went into complete remission whilst using guided imagery to combat their cancers. Another 22% experienced a decrease in the size of their tumours, and even those who died lived twice as long as they'd been expected to live. This is powerful news and hopefully will ignite you desire to study N.L.P. and hypnosis which teaches you how to consciously take control of your mind for greater success.

ENJOY YOUR LEARNING CURVE
AND KEEP COMING BACK TO BASICS

I'm sure you're amazed at how many wonderful ideas and concepts you've learned throughout RAW PERFECTION, but how many are you going to implement into your life? Remember, there will be times when you make mistakes and find it challenging, but this isn't a big deal, so don't treat it like one. Lighten up – It's all well and fine wanting to be perfect over night, but it's not necessarily the best route to take. Develop your own learning curve and you'll build references for your exciting future.

THE ULTIMATE CHALLENGE

Optimal nutrition is an excellent gateway to a rich, more fullfilling life, but health is more than just nutrition. You aren't just a bundle of cells crying out for nutrients, you are a spiritual being. For you to tap into your limitless potential, you need to be 'alive' and 'vibrating' with energy! Your bioelectrical nature must be fed with foods that have 'high vibrations' allowing your energy to grow. Green leafy vegetables, raw plant fats, fruits, vegetables, sprouts and wheatgrass juice accelerate the electrical activity inside every cell. A diet of bread, potatoes, meats, canned vegetables, and other refined 'recreational' foods doesn't!

Many people think they can supply all the nutrients necessary for peak performance by taking a standard multi-vitamin and mineral formula, but how can these kinds of supplements add life and energy to your body? A vitamin pill won't sprout up and grow into a healthy living plant! Vitamin supplements may be useful to balance an existing problem, but live raw foods create unshakeable health! Raw foods are a virtual goldmine of every conceivable nutrient needed for life. Your cells reach out for these kinds of charged nutrients with an irresistible magnetism.

I PRAY YOU CONTINUE TO DREAM
AND ACT ON THOSE DREAMS

We have journeyed a long way together. How much further you go will be down to you! RAW PERFECTION has shared with you the necessary tools and insights to radically change your life. But what you do from here is entirely your decision. When you put this book down, you can do what many people do and completely forget what you've learned and wonder why you can't get control of your life, or you can make it your personal mission to use RAW PERFECTION for what it was meant to be: A guide to living an extra-ordinary life. Make your decision wisely!

A QUICK REVIEW TO CATAPULT YOU INTO ACTION

Let's review the key concepts of RAW PERFECTION that make it such a revolutionary approach to nutrition and peak performance. You know that food has more effect on your body than any prescription drug and that cooked food is dead food! You've learned how to make the most effective use of chlorophyll-rich green leafy vegetables. Whether you juice, blend or eat more of them, you'll want them to form the foundation of your diet.

You've learned about the importance of sprouts and you've learned why it's critical to soak all nuts and seeds before eating them to disable any enzyme inhibitors. You also know that raw plant fats help eliminate cravings, whilst saturating your body with vital nutrients. Remember, raw plant fats HEAL, cooked fats KILL!

You've learned that detoxification is a process that can be accelerated with the principles of RAW PERFECTION. You've also learnt that colonic hydrotherapy is critical, especially if you've been eating a diet full of cooked food. Regardless of your health, you'll want to have one or more colonics twice a year in order to fully cleanse your colon and restore any lost vitality. Finally, section one offered you a prescription for aerobic exercise that'll help you increase your fitness and longevity.

Next you learned about fat storage and fat mobilisation and the two master hormones of energy metabolism, insulin and glucagon. You know that protein (preferably raw sources) will help stimulate the hormone glucagon and help you eliminate any unwanted fat from your body. Once you use food to control insulin and glucagon you take your health to a whole new level. You've also been introduced to the power of the super-hormones: eicosanoids. You've learned how to keep the eicosanoid production pathway functioning optimally by keeping delta 6 desaturase active, delta 5 desaturase inactive and by keeping insulin and glucagon balanced. You also discovered the magic formula for becoming an all-powerful raw-foodist by balancing chlorophyll-rich greens, raw plant fats, fruits, sprouts and vegetables to optimise eicosanoid balance.

You've learned how to use exercise as a controller of hormones, whilst unleashing the powerful human growth hormone necessary for youth enhancement. You've discovered the importance of keeping your blood sugar levels balanced before and during a workout and you know what foods are necessary for replenishing your muscles after a workout.

You've learned that stress is a powerful destroyer of health, and that the stress hormone cortisol is directly linked to high blood-insulin levels. You've learned how the hormones related to stress, nutrition and exercise all inter-relate and how Transcendental Meditation and mind-machines can help control and eliminate the stress response, whilst conditioning peak performance states of mind. You've also learned that stimulation and an enriched environment is the only way to maintain a powerful brain long into your future and that movement/exercise is a critical nutrient for increasing mental health and longevity.

You've discovered which foods balance the neurotransmitters in your brain, and finally you've discovered how to maximise your lifespan by encompassing the principle of eating an 'optimal minimum'.

I BID YOU FAREWELL AND PRAY
THAT YOU EMBRACE THE GIFT OF LIFE

I don't expect you to master this book in a day or even a week. Give yourself time. Some things we've discussed will come easier to you than others. Remember, life has a processional effect. As you make changes in the direction of perfect health, you'll learn, grow and open the doorway for more change. The tiny changes you make, over time, usually make the biggest difference.

Treat this book as a motivating force that helps you choose a different direction in life. Imagine what would have happened if you hadn't changed your eating habits. Imagine where you'd be five, ten, fifteen years from now. By changing your eating habits by only 1 degree you take a different path in life. As you travel along this path, the change will be imperceptible to begin with, but in a few years or a decade from now, the path chosen will be completely different from the one you were on, until there's no similarity at all.

This is what RAW PERFECTION can do for you. If you learn to appreciate the power of raw food and use it to your advantage the difference you'll experience in the coming few weeks, months and years will be phenomenal. Whether you do what I do and go for the 'shot gun' approach (where you use as many of the principles as possible) or whether you make tiny changes over time, you've taken responsibility and a step in the right direction. Every action you take has an equal and opposite reaction leading you towards your ultimate destination.

My last questions to you are simple. Where are you now in your life and where are you going? Where will you be five years from now or ten years from now if you follow your current path? Are you doing what you love with people who inspire you? Or, in your own opinion, are you living a mediocre existence. Be honest and take a good look at yourself. You have the capability to be and do whatever you choose. The choices you make in life take you in specific direction. Remember, the best way to predict the future is to get a clear idea of what's happening now.

MY FINAL MESSAGE TO YOU, MY FRIEND

If you can help yourself and go on to help others with this information then I congratulate you. Helping other people achieve success and fulfil their dreams is one of the greatest gifts life can give you. I challenge you to take action and use what you've learned. Make your life a masterpiece and join the elite group of people who don't just talk the talk, but walk the walk. Become a model for excellence.

For now, I thank you for your commitment and for reading RAW PERFECTION to the end. All that you've learned has helped me in my life and hopefully will help you in yours. I hope I've inspired you to the point where you continue to look for human excellence everywhere you turn. Let RAW PERFECTION be the stepping-stone that propels you to great things, in life and in love.

THE ULTIMATE RAW PERFECTION EVALUATION:
Do you utilise the power of RAW PERFECTION on a daily basis?

APPENDIX

THE RAW PERFECTION SHOPPING LIST

FRUIT
Apples, apricots, asian pear, avocado, banana, bilberry, blackberry, blackcurrant, blood orange blueberry, breadfruit, cape gooseberry/Chinese lantern, cerimoya/custard apple, cherry, cloudberry, coconut (jelly/baby coconuts are better, available from most oriental shops), cranberry, dates, dewberry, dragon fruit, durian, figs, gooseberry, grape, grapefruit, greengage, guava ,huckleberry, jakfruit, juniper berry, kiwi fruit, kumquat, lemon, lime loganberry, lychee, mango, mangosteen, melon, mulberry, nectarine, olive, orange, papaya, passion fruit, pawpaw, peach, pear, persimmon, physalis, pineapple, plantain, plum, pomegranite, pomelo, quince, rambutan, raspberry, redcurrent, satsuma, sharon fruit, starfruit/carambola, strawberry, tamarillo, tamarind, tangerine, ugli fruit, watermelon.

VEGETABLES
Artichoke, asparagus, aubergine/eggplant, beetroot, bok choy, broad bean, broccoli, brussels sprout, cabbage, carrot, cauliflower, celeriac, celery, chinese cabbage, courgette, fennel, garden pea, green bean, haricot bean, Jerusalem artichoke, kohlrabi, leek, liquorice root, marrow, okra, parsnip, radish, rhubarb, runner bean, snow pea/ mangetout, spinach, squash, sweetcorn, sweet potato, turnip, yam.

SALAD FRUITS
Bell pepper, cucumber, tomato.

LEAFY GREENS
Beet greens, chard, chicory/endive, dandelion greens, kale, lamb's lettuce, lettuce, rocket, spinach, turnip greens.

HERBS AND WILD GREENS
Balm, basil, bay leaves, borage, burdock, chomomile, hervil, chickweed, chicory/endive, chive, comfrey leaves, common orache, coriander, dandelion, dillweed, garlic mustard, horseradish, lemongrass, lemon verbena, lovage, mallow marjoram, mint, oregano, parsley, peppermint, raspberry leaf, rosemary, sage, salad burnet, savory, sea purslane, shepherd's purse, sorrel, spearmint, tarragon, thyme, watercress, watermint, wild celery, wild garlic, yarrow.

NUTS
Almonds, beechmast, brazil nut, cashew, chestnut, hazelnut/filbert, macadamia, pecan, pine nut, pistachio, walnut.

SEEDS
Aniseed, caraway, celery, dill, fennel, fenugreek, hemp, linseed/flaxseed, poppy, pumpkin, sesame, sunflower, wheat groats.

SEEDS FOR SPROUTING
Alfalfa, brussels sprout, cabbage, clover, cress, fenugreek, garlic, kale, mustard, onion, radish, turnip.

BEANS, PULSES AND LEGUMES FOR SPROUTING
Aduki/adzuki, blackeye bean, chickpea/garbanzo bean, haricot bean, lentil, lima bean, mung beans, pea, peanut, pinto bean, Soya. NOTE: NEVER spout kidney beans, they are toxic unless cooked thoroughly).

SPICES
All spice, anise, aniseed, cardamom, cinnamon, clove, cumin, mace, nutmeg, paprika, saffron, turmeric.

STIMULANTS
Cayenne pepper, chilli, Chinese five spice (cinnamon, cloves, fennel seed, star anise, and peppercorns), curry powder (up to 20spices), garlic, ginger, jalapeno pepper, onion, pepper, shallot, spring onion/scallion.

DRIED FRUITS
Apple, apricot, cherry, cranberry, currant, date, fig, mango, mulberry, peach, pineapple, prune, raisin, redcurrant, sultana.

SEA VEGETABLES
Arame, carragheen/irish moss, dulse, hiziki/hijiki, kelp/kombu, laver, nori, sea palm, wakame.

ALGAE
Chlorella, Klamath Lake blue green algae, Spirulina.

CREATIVITY – V – MONOTONY
WHAT'S THE BEST APPROACH TO RAW PERFECTION?

Ironically, both are as important as each other. Each of us has about ten favourite meals. What are yours? Do they build health or do they destroy health? It's your mission to get creative, eliminate your old favourites and replace them with 10 new meals that are in alignment with the principles of RAW PERFECTION. It is then and only then, you can use monotony to your advantage by not complicating your food choices. You'll have predictable yet enjoyable meals that serve your unassailable health. Too much diversity means you'll struggle to stick to any plan. It's your responsibility to find out what works for you. I suggest you buy 'Shazzie's detox delights' by Sharon Holdstock and fall in love with every one of her delicious raw food recipes and prepare for multiple tastegasms!

In Ragnar Berg's food analysis table you can see which foods are acid-forming (producing mucus in the body), and which foods are acid-binding (neutralising acids, helping to eliminate unwanted mucus). As you can see, olives, soybeans, figs and spinach are all incredibly powerful from this point of view, showing a high percentage of the alkaline mineral salts necessary to neutralise acidity from acid-forming foods. Not all fruits and vegetables are listed.

NAME OF FOOD	ACID-BINDING	ACID-FORMING
Most meats		9.90 – 38.61
Eggs		11.61
Cereals		2.66 – 17.96
ROOT VEGETABLES	ACID-BINDING	ACID-FORMING
White potatoes	5.90	
Sweet potatoes	10.31	
Celery roots	11.33	
Red Beets	11.37	
White turnips	10.80	
Sugar beets	9.37	
Black radish, with skin	39.40	
Horse radish, with skin	3.06	
Young radish	6.05	
Cabbages	4.02	
Red cabbage	2.20	
Endives	14.51	
Lettuce head	14.12	
Rhubarb	8.93	
Spinach	28.01	
Asparagus	1.01	
Artichoke	4.31	
Chicory	2.33	
Tomatoes	13.67	
Pumkins	.28	
Watermelon	1.83	
Cucumbers	13.50	
Red onions	1.09	
Kohlrabe root	5.99	
Cauliflowers	3.04	
Brussel sprouts		13.15
Dandelion	17.52	
Dill	18.36	
Leeks	11.00	
Watercress	4.98	

	ACID-BINDING	ACID-FORMING
String beans	8.71	
Green peas	5.15	
Dried peas		3.41
Beans, dried		9.70
Lentils		17.80
FRUITS	ACID-BINDING	ACID-FORMING
Apples	1.38	
Pears	3.26	
Plums	5.80	
Apricots	4.79	
Peaches	5.40	
Cherries	2.57	
Sour cherries	4.33	
Sweet cherries	2.69	
Dates, dried	5.50	
Figs	27.81	
Grapes	7.15	
Raisons	15.10	
Rasperries	5.19	
Oranges	9.61	
Lemons	9.90	
Pomegranates	4.15	
Pineapple	3.59	
Banana	4.38	
Olives	30.56	
Prunes	5.80	
Strawberries	1.76	
Currants	4.43	
Blackberries	7.14	
Tangerines	11.77	
NUTS	ACID-BINDING	ACID-FORMING
Walnuts		9.225
Coconut	4.09	
Hazelnut		2.08
Peanuts		16.39
Almonds		2.19
Chestnuts		9.62
GRAIN	ACID-BINDING	ACID-FORMING
Soy beans	26.58	
Rye flour		.72
Oat flour		8.08
Oat flakes		20.71

GLYCEMIC INDEX TABLE

Low Glycemic (Less than 50)	Medium Glycemic (Between 50 and 80)	High Glycemic (Greater than 80)

Grain-based foods

Low Glycemic	Medium Glycemic	High Glycemic
27 Rice bran	54 Pasta, star white, boiled 5 min.	81 Pastry
45 Barley (pearled)	58 Rice, polished, boiled 5 min	81 Wild Rice
38 Pasta, spaghetti, protein enriched	61 Spaghetti	83 Rice, white
45 Spaghetti, white, boiled 5 min	63 Wheat kernels	87 Porridge oats
46 Fettuccine.	64 Macaroni, white, boiled 5 min	87 Hamburger bun
48 Rye	68 Bread, rye pumpernickel	89 Bread, rye, whole meal
	68 Oat bran bread	92 Semolina bread
	69 Multi grain bread	92 Macaroni & Cheese
	74 Buckwheat	93 Couscous
	75 Bulger bread	95 Bread, rye, crispbread
	77 Special K	95 Barley flour bread
	78 Oat bran cereal	95 Gnocchi
	79 Brown Rice	96 Muesli
		97 Taco shells
		98 Shredded wheat

Fruits

Low Glycemic	Medium Glycemic	High Glycemic
10 Nopal (prickly pear)	53 Apples	98 Cornmeal
32 Cherries	55 Plum	100 Tortilla, corn
34 Plum	58 Pears	100 Most breads
36 Grapefruit	59 Apple juice	100 Melba Toast
40 Peaches	60 Fresh peach	103 Bagel
44 Apricots	63 Orange	103 Millet
49 Strawberries	66 Pineapple juice	109 Weetabix
	66 Grapes	115 Cornflakes
	69 Grapefruit juice	125 Rice, instant
	74 Orange juice	
	75 Kiwi	

Fruits

80 Mango
84 Banana
91 Raisins
93 Cantaloupe
94 Pineapple
103 Watermelon

Vegetables

Low Glycemic	Medium Glycemic	High Glycemic
20 Soy beans, dried	54 Brown beans	88 Beet
22 Soy beans, canned	55 Pinto beans	100 Potato, mashed
32 Dried peas	57 Haricot (navy) beans	107 Pumpkin
37 Red lentils	59 Black-eyed beans	109 Broad beans
43 Black beans	60 Baked beans (canned)	117 Cooked carrots
45 Kidney beans	65 Green peas, frozen	118 Potato, instant
46 Blackeye peas	65 Romano Beans	128 Potato, Russet, baked
46 Butter beans	68 Green peas	139 Cooked parsnips
47 Rye kernels	70 Potato, sweet	
49 Chick peas	74 Yam	
50 Green peas, dried	74 Canned kidney beans	
50 Lima beans	80 Potato, new, boiled	
	80 Sweet corn	

Dairy products	Dairy products	Snacks
46 Skim milk	52 Yoghurt	86 Cheese pizza
48 2% milk	71 Low fat ice cream	88 Muffins
49 Whole milk	87 Ice cream	91 plain crackers
20 Low fat yoghurt with SS		92 Short bread
47 Low fat yoghurt fruit		95 Angel food cake
sweetened		95 Cookies, Ryvita
43 Soy milk		96 Croissant
		97 Mars bar
		98 Crumpet
Snacks	**Snacks**	99 Corn chips
20 Peanuts	77 Crisps	108 Donut
	78 Biscuits	109 Waffles
	79 Popcorn	115 Puffed rice cakes
		116 Pretzels
		126 Honey
Simple Sugars	**Simple Sugars**	**Simple Sugars**
31 Fructose	65 Lactose	92 Sucrose
		138 glucose
		152 maltose

The glycemic index is a ranking of foods based on their immediate effect on blood glucose (blood sugar) levels. Carbohydrate foods that breakdown quickly during digestion have the highest glycemic indexes. Their blood sugar response is fast and high aggravating insulin. Carbohydrates that breakdown slowly, releasing glucose gradually into the blood stream and have low glycemic indexes.

The golden rule is to remember that you shouldn't evaluate all foods on their glycemic index rating alone. Many raw foods with a high rating are also high in vitamins, minerals, enzymes, essential fats etc. and are teeming with goodness. Use this table as just a guide and to add to your ever-growing fountain of knowledge.

USEFUL CONTACTS

Rather than list endless contacts, here are the ones that will kick-start your quest for a richer more fulfilling life. By visiting the various websites, you can begin to search out other links depending on your specific interest.

www.rawperfection.co.uk
Having read the book, you must now visit the website!

www.shazzie.com
This is one of the best websites in the world. Read Shazzie's raw story, buy her book and find yourself inspired to make the necessary changes that automatically lead to a wonderful life. See her amazing transformation photos and check out how bendy she is. Yoga will set you free!

www.fresh-network.com
The FRESH Network
P.O. Box 71
Ely
Cambridgeshire
CB7 4GU
Tel: 0870 8007070
Fax: 0870 800 7071
e-mail: info@fresh-network.com
Karen Knowler is one of the worlds leading experts in dealing with the practical and emotional aspects of transitioning from a cooked diet to a raw diet. She runs the FRESH Network and is the co-author of 'Feelgood Food'. The FRESH network can supply almost all of your needs from books, tapes, videos to sprouting equipment, juicers, dehydrators and starter kits – phone them today!

www.lifetools.com
Chris Payne is one of the most inspirational men on the planet. He has set up the worlds finest mail-order company designed to supply you with all your peak-performance needs from mind machines to photoreading. Visit the Lifetools website today.

The Colonic International Association
16 Drummond Ride
Tring
Hertfordshire
HP23 5DE

Contact the Colonic Internation Association and find out where your nearest colonic irrigation specialist resides.

www.rawfood.com
Nature's First Law
P.O. Box 900202
San Diego
CA 92190
USA
Tel: 001 619 229 8259
e-mail: nature@rawfood.com

www.egoscue.com
This website will give you access to a variety of tools that can help you realign your body and create exceptional postural health.

The Durian Fruit Centre
The Oriental City
Ground floor carpark Unit 1
No.399 Edgeware Road
Colindale
London NW9 OJJ

If you are looking for durians and young coconuts, or any other exotic fruit, take a trip to The Oriental City. Any questions, phone Alex & Felicia on 07904955716 or 07958166657.

www.takecontrol.tv
I dedicated this book to Alan Austin-Smith because without his help and belief in me, you probably wouldn't be holding this book in your hands. Alan created a revolutionary program for personal development called Take Control. If you go on one personal development program this year, go on this one.

www.centerpointe.com
This website will allow you to purchase The End Personal Development
Program that I rave about in chapter 12.

www.mckennabreen.com
I trained in N.L.P. and hypnosis with Paul McKenna, Michael Breen and
Richard Bandler. I highly recommend their trainings.

www.tonyrobbins.com
I first attended the 'Fear into Power – Firewalk experience' on my 18th
birthday and less than 10 years later I believe I've written one of the
most comprehensive nutritional/health books in existence. It all started
here. Anthony Robbins' seminars will blow you away.

INDEX